YES! YOU WILL BE A GOOD MOM!

THE 9-STEP GUIDE TO A HAPPY, POSITIVE, AND
WORRY-FREE PREGNANCY FOR FIRST TIME
MOMS AND NEW PARENTS

KELLY PRESTON, M.A.

For My Valued Readers!

3 Gifts Just for YOU

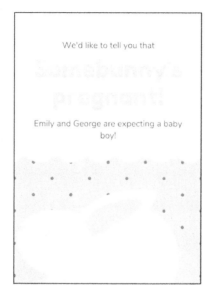

GIFT #1 I would love to give you a **FREE** completely personalized digital full-color pregnancy announcement, so you can share your exciting news!

To choose from one of **17** cute announcements visit:

https://rebrand.ly/free-pregnancy-announcement

Or use this scannable QR code:

*Scan code to choose your free personalized
pregnancy announcement.*

Pregnancy Resource Pack

Daily Journal Template

Meal Planner

Birth Plan Planner

GIFT #2 To receive your pregnancy resource pack, please visit:

https://rebrand.ly/pregnancy-resources

Or use this scannable QR code:

Scan code to receive your pregnancy resource pack.

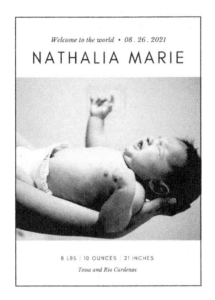

Welcome to the world • 08 . 26 . 2021

NATHALIA MARIE

8 LBS | 10 OUNCES | 21 INCHES
Tessa and Rio Cardenas

GIFT #3 Once your precious baby arrives, contact me for a **FREE** completely personalized digital birth announcement, so you can share your exciting news! I want to help you celebrate - and as a bonus for me, I get to see the sweet new babies when I create the announcements!

To choose from one of **20** cute styles (3 of which are super cool video announcements!) visit:

https://rebrand.ly/free-birth-announcement

Or use this scannable QR code:

Scan code to choose your free personalized birth announcement.

The announcements will be sent only to you, and will not be used by anyone for any reason. I hope you enjoy your 3 free gifts! If you'd like to join a group of like-minded mommies-to-be, we have a great community at:

https://www.facebook.com/
groups/pregnancy101support

~ Kelly

CONTENTS

INTRODUCTION

Jane Weideman once said: "Giving birth should be your greatest achievement, not your greatest fear." How do you define your pregnancy? Finding out you're pregnant should be the most wondrous news you ever receive. It should make your heart swell with joy, but for many moms, especially new and first-time moms, pregnancy can also bring a flurry of unexpected fearfulness and anxiety. Understandable, as you're doing something you've never done before and you're about to become someone you've never been. That can be scary! However, there's no need to feel discouraged for being worried about what comes next. You just need to learn about the facts, and they will trump the fears brewing inside of you.

Pregnancy is a miraculous experience where a new life forms from the tiniest of cells. Just as a relationship between two unique people can be delicate, so can pregnancy be if you don't have some guidance on your journey. You may find yourself worrying about things that seem superficial, such as gaining too much pregnancy weight and how you'll lose it after the baby arrives. Or you might find yourself questioning your ability to be the best mother you can be for your little one. Before you know it, you even fear morning sickness, as natural as it may be. It's only a small step from this fear to worrying about whether you're eating the right foods for this little munchkin growing inside of you.

Before long, you're stressing about stressing, and it starts going downhill from there. If there was ever a time that your brain overworks itself, it's while you're pregnant. It doesn't matter if you were healthy before pregnancy. You still find yourself worried that you'll be diagnosed with gestational diabetes or high blood pressure. What would happen to your precious baby if that happened? How could you control it? Why is the sky not bluer today? Questions come flooding as your mind works overtime.

Some moms-to-be have anxiety about the worst-case scenarios. They wonder if they'll have a miscarriage or whether their baby will be born with poor health. You start hearing words like c-section, preterm labor, and stillbirth everywhere, and you feel sure that something's going to ruin your perfect pregnancy. Your astonishingly sharp attention latches onto everything you hear that makes your worry worse. Humans are programmed to believe the negative far more easily than they believe the positive. You might then find yourself worried about labor itself. Will you make it to the hospital on time? Will your water break in public? Will the pain be as unbearable as the screams you hear in the movies? And just like that, your joyful journey turns into a worry-filled pregnancy.

How can you enjoy this incredible gift if there's so much to worry about? The first thing you need to know is just how common these fears can be, even though the negative outcomes are very unlikely to happen to you. Unlikely is the key word here. We tend to amplify our attention on the things that *could* go wrong, instead of enjoying every moment with our developing babies. An interesting six-month study was published in *Frontiers in Psychology* (Vismara et al., 2016). The study focused on first-time expectant mothers and fathers, and the results proved how normal it is if you're anxious. Not only were first-time parents more anxious about their journey, but they also showed increased anxiety as new parents after their babies were born. So, you're not alone in this worry boat, but you don't need to be there. You can jump out any time.

Gentle and evidence-based guidance can help you understand why your fears stir during a time that should be joyous and exciting. It can also show you just how uncommon the manifestation of these fears is in the real world. Take a deep breath, and know this - fear is common, but the chances of having an unhealthy pregnancy are nearly as rare as hair growing on your gums. And yes, that's very rare! Again, you're new to this journey, and it's okay to be afraid of anything unknown. Fortunately, you're not the first mom to face these fears and anxieties.

This book will help you understand what's within your control, and how you can promote a happier, healthier, and worry-free pregnancy. This journey is yours to love, and nothing should deprive you of that. The nine steps in this guide allow you to connect deeper with your unborn baby and teach you about the most common fears in pregnancy and how you can deal with them. You'll also learn about simple, non-medicinal ways to decrease genuine risks because sometimes, people have a greater risk of complications merely because they don't know how to prevent them. You'll learn what to eat to ensure better nutrition for your baby, and this will prevent certain fears from manifesting.

You won't have to give up your entire kitchen, either. Eating right for the optimal outcome is about balancing the nutrients that promote better circulation, improved brain development for the baby, and keep your body in optimal health to carry your baby to full-term. You'll also learn about pregnancy superfoods, and how to sleep better because rest is a vital part of your journey. Everything requires balance though, and you'll discover the pregnancy-safe exercises you can use to improve your baby's well-being even more. Preparing your mind and body for what comes at the end of your journey can easily be achieved by visiting prenatal classes, which come with numerous benefits. Moreover, this book will help you find ways to connect deeper with your unborn bundle of joy because this is one thing you don't want to miss out on. You can bond with your baby before birth, and so can your co-parent.

Your pregnancy journey will only improve as you learn how to manage your anxiety levels. Fear is but an emotion. It has no face or physical space. It can be challenged, and so can your thoughts. Two of the major steps you'll take toward a happier pregnancy are to challenge and erase worrisome thoughts and unhelpful emotions. Building your inner strength and resilience will help you overcome any worries that stop you from having the pregnancy you deserve. You're about to realize that you can be prepared for anything, expect nothing, and overcome everything. You've got this!

People often ask me why I love to help others have a happy pregnancy and calm parenting, and I always return to the same answer. My husband and I struggled with infertility for years, and that made us appreciate the journey from a different perspective. We required medical intervention to welcome our babies, and today, we have two healthy children, a boy, and a girl. I won't deny the fact that fear was an intricate part of our journey and it felt exacerbated by the struggle we had to become parents. Most newly pregnant moms have worries crawl into their minds, and I was no different. This only made my pregnancy a fearful challenge, instead of the precious experience I wanted to enjoy. The ball was in my court though. I had a decision to make.

I could either be overwhelmed by my fears, or I could learn, research, and find answers to my most pressing questions. Sadly, researching can sometimes exaggerate our fears, especially if we rely on "Dr. Google". Sometimes we only read the nonsense that exaggerates the worries more. At the end of the day, this only steals your pregnancy contentment and connection to the baby, while providing you with information that has little value. Instead, I chose to research credible facts because that's what I learned to do during my post-secondary education and in my line of work. I have a Master's Degree in clinical psychology, focusing on children.

I worked for many years in the psychological services department of a large school board, working with various schools and hundreds of children. Decreasing worry and changing what can be changed has helped many of the children with whom I work. I also have a large mom's support group now, and we encourage each other to be happy and connected with our babies. Experience is one thing that can't be dismissed, and I can guide you from both a professional and motherly background. The only thing that genuinely matters right now is that you turn a fearful pregnancy into one filled with joy and connectedness. Whatever your doubts may be, and whatever fears stand in your way, you can overcome them.

You must ask yourself whether you want your pregnancy to be filled with fear and worry or to be your most magnificent accomplishment? I think you know the answer, and this guide will help you get there.

STEP 1: YOU'RE NOT ALONE!
EDUCATION IS REVELATION

*P*regnancy fears are common, especially among first-time moms. The thought of welcoming your bundle of joy into this world can be overwhelmingly exciting, but the fears can be just as intense. The truth is that most moms and babies come out of the delivery room healthy, and the original fears are often created by a lack of education. Speculating about something always conjures much worse imaginings than educating yourself about it. It also doesn't help that many mothers share their horror stories which make you more anxious. If you can remove the speculation and replace it with facts, you will be far less fearful and worried. Education is the first important step as a new mom-to-be, and it removes guesses and speculations that make your journey less enjoyable, and more fearful than it should be.

Common Worries and Why They Don't Need to Be

First-time moms are overwhelmed with fears about pregnancy, but facts put the guesses to rest. Let's discuss which are the most common fears during pregnancy and what the truth is behind them.

Morning Sickness

Morning sickness has a way of conjuring fears that shouldn't be part of your exciting journey. It's not that newly pregnant moms are worried about the morning sickness itself, but more that they are concerned that it will prevent the baby from getting the nutrients it needs. Since it's most common in the first trimester, one thing you should realize is that your baby is incredibly small during this stage of development, and they don't need much nutrition. In fact, just staying hydrated gives your baby much of what they need to grow. Don't worry about being sick for fear that your baby is not getting what it needs, as they'll get what nutrition they require from whatever you can manage to eat. Fortunately, morning sickness starts fading between 12 and 16 weeks, but you can visit your doctor if you're losing weight unintentionally.

If you are suffering from morning sickness, there are a few tricks you can use to help alleviate it. Eat a small snack at bedtime, and munch on crackers or pretzels before getting out of bed in the morning. Not having an empty stomach can reduce nausea. When your stomach is turning too much, start your day with water to hydrate first. Sometimes adding a bit of lemon to your water can help. Switch to eating six mini-meals instead of three large ones, and snack on something small every two hours if you can't manage a meal. Eating bland foods like crackers, rice cakes, toast, bread, rice, potatoes, and pretzels can soothe morning sickness. Avoid onions, garlic, spicy or strong smelling foods, citrus juices, milk or caffeinated drinks.

Sometimes, we develop food aversions where we feel sick when certain foods are eaten (or even smelled). If you suffer from this, substitutions can be made to make sure you still get maximum nutrition each day. For meat, you can eat tofu, beans, nuts, and soy. For milk, you can switch to almond milk, cheese, yogurt, and drinks fortified with calcium and vitamin D.

Switch your vegetables to fruit if you need to. Bananas filled with potassium are a great option.

Eating the Wrong Foods

Moms-to-be also worry about what they eat, and whether something they have eaten might harm the baby. Eating and drinking the right stuff during pregnancy certainly makes a difference in the way you feel, what you can expect, and how healthy you and your baby will be. Some food items are discouraged like caffeine and fish that are high in mercury content, and there are definitely foods that aren't good for your baby's development. However, education is the way to put this worry to rest. Knowing what to eat, and what not to eat, will effectively alleviate this stressor. Eating properly is a huge part of a healthy pregnancy and baby, and you'll learn more about it in step two.

Gaining Too Much Weight (and Being Unable to Lose it!)

Weight gain during pregnancy also leads to a few concerns for moms-to-be. Will you be able to lose it? Will you gain too much? Unfortunately, some women do gain more than they should, but being aware of this dilemma means you're already keeping an eye on it. Remember you aren't really eating for two, as much as some moms-to-be love using this excuse. You only need a few hundred extra calories per day for a growing baby. Pregnancy is not an excuse to eat whatever you want whenever you want. The occasional treat is fine, but food acts as fuel for you and your baby, so stick mainly to nutritious foods that offer maximum nutritional benefits. Only allow yourself to gain weight according to the standard guidelines. Educating yourself on these guidelines is the first step towards healthy weight gain. And if your weight gain is on par with the suggested amount, you won't have to worry about not being able to lose it after the baby comes!

If your body mass index (BMI) is between 20 and 25, meaning you were average weight before conceiving, you should gain between two and four pounds during the entire first trimester, and one pound for every week thereafter. This puts your total weight gain between 25- and 35-pounds during pregnancy - and don't worry, you'll drop most of the weight after delivering your bundle of joy. A great way to shed weight after giving birth is with a postnatal workout class. Sometimes, you can even bring your baby along to meet little friends, and you can meet new moms at the same time. Breastfeeding also naturally helps with weight loss, if you choose to feed your baby that way.

Crushing Baby While Sleeping

Moms also worry that they're going to crush their babies-to-be while they sleep, and this thought often feels logical to the pregnant mama. However, it's not harmful to a baby in early pregnancy if you roll onto your stomach. Your body was designed to protect your developing child. And realistically, you won't be comfortable enough to sleep on your stomach once it becomes dangerous. Imagine yourself lying on your stomach while you have a big belly. It would be like trying to sleep while balancing on a beach ball! This is not a position your body would willingly go into, even during your deepest slumber.

Stress

Stressing about stress during pregnancy is quite common, but the truth is that your baby can withstand the majority of everyday stressors. They are stronger than you think. Your baby can manage the usual work pressure and the traffic jams that have you cursing the driver in front of you. However, if the stress impairs your capacity to function at work, home, or in relationships, then you can seek ways to diminish it. Moms-to-be who manage their stress effectively have a lower chance of preterm birth, underweight babies, and behavioral issues from their kiddos. Step six of this book will help you gather tools to cope with stress so you can alleviate this worry and have a perfectly healthy baby.

Complications

Complications during pregnancy are also commonly feared, especially gestational diabetes and preeclampsia, which is gestational hypertension. Thankfully, between 92 and 95% of moms-to-be **don't** get preeclampsia, and 96% of moms-to-be don't suffer from gestational diabetes (Drelsbach, 2015). It's more common in women who already have borderline hypertension or diabetes. Preeclampsia generally shows up in the second half of your pregnancy, but in some cases, it's so late that it doesn't affect you or the baby anyway. Either way, doctors normally find signs of complications early, and they'll monitor your condition closely if you're in the very small percentage of women with these problems. Otherwise, there are some preventative measures you can take at home.

To prevent preeclampsia, you should consume more calcium, so add milk, leafy greens, fortified orange juice, sesame seeds, soy, broccoli, sardines, and canned salmon to your diet. Eating more vegetables and potassium-rich bananas can also reduce your blood pressure. Vitamin D is another blood pressure regulator, and so is chocolate. Treating yourself to five or more portions of chocolate weekly can significantly reduce the risk of preeclampsia, so hopefully, it's on your list of cravings!

Gestational diabetes can also be prevented with some simple actions and education. The first secret is to maintain a healthy weight gain during pregnancy. Track your weight daily, and keep a journal of your gains. This allows you to adjust your diet to include more nutritional foods and less non-nutritional foods if you're gaining too fast. Limit your consumption of high-starch foods as well, and use yoga or other forms of exercise to regulate your blood sugar levels better. The best way to regulate and maintain your blood sugar levels is by exercising for 30 minutes a day. Aim for five days of exercise and two days of rest, but every day is even better. Exercise is most effective if you start before 16 weeks, but if you are past that point, start now. You can also purchase a blood glucose monitor to use at home, and you should visit your doctor to test your levels between 24 and 28 weeks.

More Typical Fears During Pregnancy

There are a few more serious fears among new moms-to-be because we all want our babies to be the healthiest little munchkins around. Some facts and preventative measures can improve your chances of having a stressless pregnancy.

Miscarriage

Miscarriage is a common concern in the first trimester at a time when you should be enjoying the days before your belly grows and your pants get tighter. You may be part of the 75% of concerned moms (it's a very common fear!), but miscarriage is actually an unlikely occurrence in real life (Condie, 2020). Between 88 and 90% of expectant moms have a joyful pregnancy without this fear becoming reality. Your risk decreases to only five percent once you hear your baby's heartbeat between six and eight weeks, and 99% of women won't experience miscarriage after 12 weeks. According to research by the University of Amsterdam, half of the miscarriages are due to chromosomal abnormalities and may happen before you are even aware you're pregnant (Goddijn & Leschot, 2002).

Another fear that often plagues new moms-to-be is that they might have recurrent miscarriages. We often watch movies about couples who try and try again, and this can make new moms-to-be quite nervous. According to research published in *The Lancet*, 99% of women will **not** have a second miscarriage (Rai & Regan, 2006). These figures are highly in your favor of carrying your baby to a healthy term, so the fears surrounding miscarriage are misguided by movies and the very few couples who suffer from repeated fertility issues.

Spotting can be very worrisome for newly pregnant women. What you may not realize is that 25% of women spot or bleed in the first trimester. It's always good to be safe and visit your obstetrician-gynecologist (OB-GYN), but you're not the only woman spotting if you do. In fact, it happened to me with my second child. I had light spotting and because I was breastfeeding my daughter at that time, I thought the spotting was actually very light menstruation. I didn't even realize I was pregnant until I was 18 weeks along and felt my son kicking! (Yes, I'm one of the stories that people hear about but don't believe). So don't let spotting scare you, but get it checked out to be safe.

The misconceptions about what causes miscarriages are also vast. Sex, heavy lifting, and exercise don't lead to miscarriages, but some habits could trigger the worst-case scenario, and this is why education is so vital. Caffeine isn't good for pregnant moms. Drinking two or more cups of coffee or tea daily could raise your risk, but drinking less than six fluid ounces of coffee is safe if you need the kickstart. Research by the Imperial College School of Medicine in London has highlighted some other triggers (Regan & Rai, 2000). Chronic conditions like thyroid disease and diabetes should be kept under control for the safest pregnancy in the first trimester. Diabetics have no greater risk for miscarriage if their condition is under control, so speak to your doctor and maintain your blood glucose levels as best you can.

Smoking is another cause for concern, especially in the first trimester, and drinking is not advised, either. Even three alcoholic drinks per week during the first 10 weeks could make your chances of having a successful first-trimester decrease. And needless to say, using drugs can place you in the rare category of miscarriage. To give your baby everything they need to develop correctly in the first trimester, you should avoid drinking, smoking, and using drugs. You should also start taking a multivitamin for expectant mothers, and you should cut down your caffeine intake. Otherwise, you're doing just fine because the risk factors are low.

Birth Defects

Birth defects are also commonly feared. For some reason, we worry our children will look like aliens when they exit the womb. The fear of birth defects is a strong contender among women who've never had kids before, and an unchecked imagination can be a very powerful enemy. Not to mention how your grandmother now insists on telling you every genetic disorder that runs in the family, even though you're perfectly healthy. People don't always stop to think before they speak to new moms-to-be. Birth defects aren't something we like discussing, but it falls under the umbrella of possibilities, so it becomes a valid fear. Rest easy, though. Even though 78% of new moms worry about birth defects, the fact is that 97% of babies are born with all their little toes and fingers in the right places (Tarkan, 2018). Odds are overwhelmingly in your favor!

America is a first-world country, and the healthcare system combined with technology has allowed us to test for most defects before birth. Even the minor defects babies are rarely born with, such as a clubbed foot, heart defect, or webbed toes are easily treatable with surgery. Many heart defects successfully correct themselves, and no surgery is even required. And remember, 97% of babies are born perfectly healthy. This statistic is one worth repeating.

Birth defects are also easy to prevent if you're following educated advice. The best prevention is to pretend you're pregnant from the moment you plan to conceive. Stop drinking, smoking, and using drugs. Even prescription drugs and herbal/natural supplements should be discussed with your physician. You should control diabetes if you have it, drop some pounds if you're overweight, prevent chemical exposure, and avoid the Zika virus. If you must enter areas known for the Zika virus, be sure to use pregnancy-safe bug spray.

Start taking enough folic acid daily to prevent neural tube birth defects. An amount of 600 micrograms (mcg) daily will do the trick. If you don't like supplements, you can eat enough folic acid by adding spinach, beans, milk, bananas, peas, or dark green vegetables like kale and broccoli to your diet. Folic acid is also found in enriched grain foods like bread, pasta, and cereal.

You should also remove bisphenol A (BPA) plastics in your home. Plastic products with the recycle symbols three, six, and seven contain phthalates, which can interfere with the development of your baby. Don't be spooked if you've been using them, but get rid of what you can now, and minimize your exposure going forward. They normally only pose a problem once heated, but you can minimize your contact with them anyway.

Premature Labor

Premature labor is another common concern among moms-to-be. As many as 71% of moms fear preterm birth, but the good news is that 88% of babies are born full-term (Tarkan, 2018). Most babies are born after 37 weeks gestation, which makes them full-term bloomers. Of the babies who are born preterm, most are only a few days or weeks early, so don't let the 12% of early arrivers scare you. My daughter was born 1 day before 37 weeks, but that means she was counted as preterm! What many moms-to-be also need to understand is that babies can survive and thrive after only 24 weeks gestation. Your baby is a fighter, and they have a **much** higher chance of being born within the late term than they do in the early term. Moreover, 30% of early labor incidents stop on their own without medical intervention. Early labor that doesn't stop on its own can be successfully halted by your physician. As with any potential risk, there are a few simple ways you can best avoid this complication, and that's where education again comes in.

Some ways to increase your chance of delivering a full-term baby are to stop smoking, drinking, and using drugs that aren't pregnancy-safe. You can ask your OB-GYN what drugs you should avoid as they know your individual needs. Blood sugar and blood pressure should also be monitored closely for a longer-term pregnancy, and periodontal diseases should be addressed promptly. Healthier gums and teeth are known to assist your pregnancy duration, so keep them clean, and visit your dentist when you have problems. Infections, big and small, must be addressed hastily to prolong the time your baby has to develop inside the womb. Don't allow infections to get out of control.

Two highly enjoyable practices promote a full-term birth as well. Meditation calms the mind and body, allowing your baby to feel as peaceful as you. The *Journal of Bodywork and Movement Therapies* published research that showed that yoga was used to increase the likelihood of full-term labor (Mooventhan, 2019). Yoga for moms-to-be is an exciting way to extend your pregnancy term, but it also does so much more, which you'll learn about in step five. These are just a number of ways you can decrease the risk of premature birth.

Stillbirth

Stillbirth must be the most devastating fear that plagues moms-to-be, but it can also cause unregulated anxiety that isn't necessary. According to the Centers for Disease Control and Prevention (CDC, 2020), 99.4% of births are live and the babies cry their little lungs out. 99.4%! It's a minute risk you shouldn't be obsessing about during pregnancy. Late stillbirths that happen between 28 and 36 weeks, and term stillbirths that happen after 37 weeks are extremely rare, so rather focus on prevention instead of worries. Avoiding cigarettes can decrease the risks involved. It's not a surprise that smoking is risky for many of the fears described in this step, so quitting is the best thing you can do for yourself and your baby.

Uncontrolled diabetes and hypertension can also be dangerous. The key here is the word 'uncontrolled,' so keeping your thumb on these conditions can improve your chance of having a healthy, crying baby. Sleeping on your back in later pregnancy is also not advised. Sleeping on your side can reduce stillbirth risk by 50% (Ross-White, 2017). Sleeping on the left side when further along in your pregnancy can help you and your baby remain healthier by improving the blood flow to your heart, kidneys, and uterus. It also prevents the uterus from pressing against your liver. Moreover, there's better blood flow to the baby, and your little one can receive the nutrients and oxygen they need. Both of you will be much healthier.

Labor Concerns

Labor has been painted as a nightmarish scene by the people who've done it and in the movies we binge-watch, but educating yourself about what can be expected and what shouldn't be feared is a great way to soothe your concerns about the birthing process. Believe me, your speculation about the process is probably much more horrific than the actual event. Learning all you can in advance can alleviate many of your labor worries.

Water Breaking

Some women worry about their water breaking in public. This is another notion made famous by comedies and dramas, but the slippery floor that sends passers-by on a ski trip doesn't happen very often, if at all. The sack of amniotic fluid that surrounds your baby normally breaks after your labor begins and hardly ever before contractions. Contractions start before the water breaks in 90 to 92% of women (Marcin & Nwadike, 2020). So, you'll most likely have a warning before the splash. In many cases, the doctor has to break your water!

Delivering in a Taxi

Another concern about labor is that you won't make it to the hospital on time, which is only aggravated by the movies showing moms giving birth in cabs. Movies sure are a bad way to educate yourself!

Babies don't just pop out of the womb like a jack in the box. It's a very slow process where mom goes through various stages, and chances are that you'll be in labor for hours before this happens. A huge study by the Neonatal Unit at Marston Green Hospital in England proved just how rare this occurrence is (Bhoopalam & Watkinson, 1991). The hospital shared records of how many moms made it to the hospital before giving birth, and more than 99% of the 31,000 moms safely gave birth in the comfort of the hospital over the course of five years. With there being an average of eight hours for the active stage of labor, first-time moms have lots of time to get to the hospital. The best way to calm your nerves about this fear is to prepare. Make sure you have pre-packed a bag for hospital day and plan your route, as well as your driver beforehand. Preparation is the key to having enough time in case you're a lucky lady who delivers fast on her first go.

Labor Itself

Another fear moms-to-be often have is about the labor process itself. Even some of the bravest women worry about the pain of labor. We tend to develop preconceptions of what labor will entail for us based on those dreaded movies again (so much screaming!)

and horror stories from women who relish feeding our fears. A majority of the stories we are told are negative because humans have a negative bias and often see the worst in everything. Many labor stories aren't horror stories, though. I should tell you about a good friend of mine. 'Jess' is the one and only woman I know who slept through labor. The nurses tried on numerous occasions to wake her up, but she fell asleep again and again until her daughter entered this world.

One thing we can't do is guess what labor will be like for us as individuals, and the speculation is almost always worse than the reality. Every woman experiences labor differently, and every baby is unique. To avoid disappointment and "fear-mongering", you must ask people to stop telling you stories. Their labor won't be your labor, so there's no point hearing their horror stories.

The best way to set your expectations is to educate yourself about the various options for labor and pain management. Don't imagine Jess's story as your own. She's part of an exclusive and rare club. And don't expect yourself to manage the pain the same way your sister did, especially if she broke her husband's hand. Your expectations must be yours alone, and knowing what options you have when the time comes will allow you to give informed consent for all aspects of delivery. It removes the guesswork, which is vital to alleviating fears about the unknown.

Be prepared for any outcome by choosing your own labor team, which is made of people with similar goals for your optimal birth. Where you have your baby, and how you deal with the pain is up to you. Involve your partner, and make a birth plan. But be aware that the plan can change during labor, and that doesn't mean you failed. Last-minute changes only indicate that you want the safest birth for you and your baby, and you will do what is necessary to achieve that. Ultimately, it's your baby who's in charge of what happens next. Find out about the different options you may have to switch to beforehand so you can give educated consent to what must happen. This allows you to still stay in some control, and you won't have to make quick decisions at a moment when your mind is focused on your labor. Learn about pain management options in advance also – even if you aren't intending to use any medication. Epidurals are a lot safer for you and the baby nowadays, so understand what may happen if you need one during labor. Epidurals don't prolong the longer stage of labor. That's a myth. It may prolong the pushing, but this is a short stage anyway.

Sign up for Lamaze or other prenatal classes, or enlist a birthing doula or coach to prepare you for labor. Knowing why the pain exists can help you ease anxiety and focus on your breathing. There are non-medicinal pain relief options like labor in a bath, hypnobirthing, and changing positions. But if these aren't cutting it, the last thing you want is to have to learn about pain relief options while you're in pain. So again, learn all your options in advance. You may change your mind during labor, even if you opted for no pain relief in your birthing plan. Education will naturally alleviate many of the concerns you have about labor.

Who Let the Poop Out?

Another common labor fear is that you'll poop while delivering. Somehow no one really talks about this fear. You might assume that I'm going to tell you that it doesn't happen. In fact, it happens more often than the horror story moms like to admit, but it's actually a really good thing. No, this is not a crazy statement. Pooping while pushing is a good indicator that the baby's about to come, so doctors actually welcome it!

In fact, they are excited about it! Pooping on the delivery table means things are coming along naturally, including your baby. It also means that a c-section will not be necessary.

C-Section

A c-section is another fear for moms-to-be, but they are mostly planned. An emergency c-section is uncommon, and if it happens, you and your baby will likely come out of surgery healthy and happy. The most stressful part of the potential for a c-section is when it's a last-minute decision, and you aren't sure of the pros and cons. It's important to educate yourself about the reasons why c-sections are necessary in some cases and familiarize yourself with the procedure so that you can decide from an informed perspective if the need arises. In most cases, the baby is too large, the baby is breech, or there's an issue with the placenta. In these circumstances, it's safer for you and your baby to have a c-section, and thank goodness we have the technology for this. Imagine giving birth in the 1800s?

Anyway, I found myself in the position of needing an unplanned c-section. When I went into labor with my first child, the doctor realized that she was lying transverse, not head down. So in essence, she was lying sideways across my pelvis. Though he tried to manipulate her to move into position, she was stubborn (still is!) and continued lying transverse. If we went ahead with natural labor, she would have been forced to come out bum first, which obviously wouldn't be great. We were informed that a c-section would be the safest option, and knowing that it would be best for the baby (and myself) we went ahead. Well, as it turned out, there was actually a "true knot" in the umbilical cord. And yes, it is precisely as it sounds. Somehow during all her flipping and twisting in utero, she managed to put a knot in the umbilical cord. Now, this was no big deal, because I had a c-section. However, if I'd delivered her naturally there was a chance that the knot would have tightened and cut off her circulation. My c-section was a blessing in disguise! Even still, at the time it was a bit alarming because I hadn't thought to educate myself in advance. I don't want you to make the same mistake.

Stages of Labor

Educating yourself about the three stages of labor can also calm your mind, and lessen your worries about giving birth.

The first stage is called early and active labor. Early labor is the longest stage, and it can last up to 24 hours for first-time moms. Your contractions will last about 60 seconds, and they'll be between five and 30 minutes apart. Your doctor will advise you in advance about when to arrive at the hospital. Generally, you'll call your doctor to meet you at the hospital if you have contractions less than five minutes apart for about an hour. You'll be in active labor if you start bleeding or your water breaks, or when your contractions become stronger and last longer, up to about 90 seconds at two to five-minute intervals. This stage of labor can last up to eight hours for new moms.

The second stage is called transition, pushing, and birth. This is the stage when the doctor tells you to push. Your cervix is dilated to about 10 centimeters now, and you're in the home stretch. The pushing stage can last from minutes to four hours, but it's the shortest one. You'll feel the urge to push as pressure builds.

Stage three comes after your baby is born. You still need to birth the placenta, which can take between five and 60 minutes. Mild contractions will still persist during this stage.

Expect the three stages, and know that they may last this long. They may not. That's up to the little guy or girl waiting to enter this world. Having clear expectations can help reduce anxiety, and who knows? You might just be one of the lucky moms who experiences a shorter or less painful birth. Your pain tolerance differs from every other woman. Labor for you cannot be defined by what others have experienced. It can only be understood so that your expectations don't disappoint you.

After Labor Worries

Even when your baby rests safely in your arms, you can still have a few new mom fears. Heck, some women worry about these issues long before their babies arrive. One thing you should always consider is that this is a new journey for you. You're allowed to be worried, but don't allow the concerns to define you. Learn more about the facts, and you'll have control over your fears.

Breastfeeding

Breastfeeding has 60% of new moms worried, but 90% of moms are successful with it (Tarkan, 2018). The key to success is to be patient and not give up early when both you and your baby are still learning. It can take anywhere from two to three weeks for both of you to master this bonding exercise. It's not an instantaneous thing. Breastfeeding worries for moms include being bitten, tenderness, latching issues, and leaking in public. A little education can help ease these worries, however.

A baby can't physically bite your nipples when they're properly latched, and you should immediately take them off your breast when they unlatch, so they won't bite. Tenderness isn't a problem when the baby latches correctly, either. Your nipples will get used to it, and you can use lanolin cream or olive oil before and after feeding in the meantime. Latching issues can resolve in a day or two when you learn how to properly position your baby for feeding. A nurse or lactation consultant can show you how to position your baby correctly.

Being prepared in advance helps defeat breast-feeding worries. Find a lactation consultant **before** your baby arrives, so you can call them if there's an issue. Leaking in public can also be managed if you purchase breast pads beforehand. Breast pads are simply little cloth inserts you place in your bra to absorb any leaking milk. Always carry a few with you just in case. Undoubtedly, you'll find yourself breast-feeding in no time as long as you persevere.

Don't fear feeling trapped, either. So many moms have told me they are worried that breastfeeding will make them feel like a milk machine. Rest easy, as you can always use a breast pump to fill bottles when you need to go out. Prevent discomfort by planning activities around your feeding schedule if you're not pumping beforehand.

Before you know it, you'll be weaning your baby, which may actually bring a sense of loss because amazing bonding happens when you breastfeed a baby. Breastfeeding gives you uninterrupted time with your baby so the two of you can relax and connect more deeply. Even if you aren't intending to breastfeed, the bonding you will experience while feeding your baby is amazing. I still remember bottle-feeding my niece when she was only a couple of weeks old. Just that one experience alone made me love that girl to pieces!

Another fear of breastfeeding is the thought of doing it in public. There are many restrooms with nursing stations now, and you can use a nursing blanket to cover yourself up if you feel uncomfortable. You get used to feeding your baby wherever and whenever you need to. I've done it at the mall, on an airplane, and at Disney World! It's amazing how quickly it all becomes second nature.

At the end of the day, breastfeeding is a choice, and you can turn to formula if you've given it your all and it didn't work. Don't fear the judgment of others. This is your baby, and you decide what's best for him/her. Only you'll know if breastfeeding isn't working, or if it isn't right for you.

Fear of Being a Bad Mother

Worrying about the fact that you won't be a good mother may also cross your mind, but fear not! There's a natural instinct that kicks in when your baby enters this world. Firstly, if you're already thinking about being a good mother, it means you're worried about your baby's well-being. Considering your baby's well-being is what makes you research your journey ahead so that you apply the best parenting knowledge to it. All you can do is your best. Worrying about being a good mom means you understand the incredible magnitude of your role. This motivates and guides you in motherhood, and you automatically put your baby's needs first.

The maternal instinct is a genuine thing, and you'll know what your child needs and what's wrong when the time comes. Your confidence in motherhood takes time to build, but it will come with every choice you make in your baby's favor. The attachment between you will also grow from the day your child is born, if not earlier. During birth, two chemicals release into your bloodstream, namely oxytocin, and estrogen. Oxytocin is the bonding hormone, which improves your desire to parent instinctively. Estrogen will be plentiful during birth, and this improves your intuition.

If you still have worries that you won't be a great mom, try to learn from people you know who are good parents. Spend time with them, and allow yourself the time to build the confidence you need.

Irrespective of what you fear, nothing's holding you back from seeking support from friends, relatives, your partner, a midwife, or your doctor. Pregnancy should be an exciting and wondrous journey. The revelations revealed in this step have hopefully eased the pressure of many of your fears, but if not, please continue to research using credible sources, not "Dr. Google". You can never know too much when you become responsible for a miniature version of yourself. Just make sure you're not listening to tales from people who only strike fear in your heart. Pregnancy is a beautiful journey, so don't let anyone ruin it for you.

2

STEP 2: ORDER UP! NOURISHMENT FOR FLOURISHMENT

*P*regnancy is a rollercoaster of unpredictable joyous and anxious moments. Your emotions aren't the only ride you get to 'enjoy' in pregnancy. You wake up one morning with the weirdest and least rational craving as you listen to your stomach growl. You can't quite pinpoint what you crave, but you head to the kitchen anyway. Suddenly, your favorite cereal makes your stomach turn, but wait, your eyes latch onto the cardboard box. Next thing you know, you're craving paper. You can't explain this, but you're craving things that should never be eaten. Cravings aren't well understood yet, but there's one fact that remains a key to a flourishing pregnancy. What you eat is what you become, and what you consume helps determine your baby's health.

Nutritional Basics

Good nutrition can resolve many of the worries you might have. It can help manage morning sickness, alleviate the fear of eating foods that aren't good for the baby, and help you maintain healthier weight gain. You'll also lose the pregnancy weight easier after delivery. Food can also affect your emotional well-being, so you'll be stressing less about your worries if you're eating right. Eating the right stuff also reduces the risks of gestational diabetes, preeclampsia, birth defects, and preterm labor, which are all common fears. You'll also have all the nutrients your body needs for when you start breastfeeding, and you'll know you're already a good mother when you take time to consider which foods help your baby. So, nutrition is the second step of your journey.

Think for a moment about the miracle of pregnancy. Inside of you, what started as a peanut-shaped embryo will eventually develop into a living, breathing human with arms, legs, bones, organs, and the cutest smile (just you wait!). Your baby is transforming from an egg to a fully-functioning little person in a mere nine months. When you focus on the development of this tiny person inside of you, it becomes clearer that what you eat truly matters. Your nutritional choices can help your precious baby transform healthily. A high-quality diet filled with nutritionally dense foods will add to a worry-free pregnancy because you remove one of the main contributing factors to many of the feared outcomes mentioned in step one.

A good quality diet can prevent complications like gestational diabetes, preeclampsia, and birth defects. It can also reduce the risks of miscarriage when you kick alcohol, caffeine, and cigarettes to the curb. Proper nutrition also helps you lose the baby weight easier after birth, and most importantly, it can ensure proper fetal development. Beyond the advantageous hormonal regulation with better food, you'll be able to enjoy your journey into motherhood. Let's face it, pregnancy already throws your hormones around. You certainly don't want food to be on the other side of the court, slamming your hormones back and forth. Your body is a delicate ecosystem, even more so while pregnant. It houses your well-being, as well as your baby's.

Empty calories and non-nutritional foods are not top of the dietary list. We can't do anything about cravings, and we can allow ourselves a treat once in a while without guilt. It's not the end of the world if you've been eating wrong up to this point. Pregnancy diets can be confusing, but they don't need to be. Your baby only needs an additional 350 to 450 calories daily (Ben-Joseph, 2017). Understanding your weight gain recommendations will help you design your diet plan. You should aim for 25 to 35 pounds if you have an average BMI, but not all of this weight goes to your baby. This chart shows the expected weight division in pounds (lbs) during pregnancy for an average weight individual.

Amniotic fluid	2 lbs	Extra fluids	4 lbs
Baby	Roughly 7.5 lbs	Placenta	1.5 lbs
Breast enlargement	2 lbs	Stored fat, nutrients, & protein	7 lbs
Extra blood	4 lbs	Uterus enlargement	2 lbs

Vital Nutrients

The stored fats, nutrients, and proteins you gain in your pregnancy weight make up nearly as much weight as your baby before delivery. This is necessary because pregnant women require additional nutrients so the fetus or baby can absorb what's needed. Consuming foods that contain the necessary nutrients for storage and absorption will ensure that your baby has everything they need to develop healthily. The charts below indicate which nutrients you and your baby need for flourishment. It also indicates each nutrients' recommended dose and what advantages it has.

Calcium

Calcium	Strengthens bones and teeth for you and your baby.
1,000 milligrams daily	Prevents osteoporosis for you later in life.
	Allows blood to clot normally.
	Promotes stronger nerves and muscles for both of you.
	Strengthens you and your baby's heart muscles.
	Helps the baby develop healthy bones.

Calcium should be increased during pregnancy and breastfeeding. Great sources of calcium include:

- Fortified low-fat milk, cream, cheese, and yogurt;
- Broccoli, spinach, kale, bok choy, okra, mustard greens, and collards;
- Canned salmon with bones and sardines;
- Dried beans and peas;

- Calcium-fortified juice, soy milk, and tofu.

Docosahexaenoic acid **(DHA)** or **omega-3 fatty acids** 200 to 300 milligrams daily	Promotes cognitive functions in you and your baby. Improves eye and brain development in the baby. Improves your energy.

Omega-3 fatty acids can be sourced from:

- Salmon, sardines, and light tuna;
- Olive, sunflower, avocado, and peanut oil;
- Nuts and seeds.

Fiber 30 grams daily	Keeps your bowel movements regular. Prevents constipation. Reduces your risk of hemorrhoids.

Your fiber intake should increase slowly during pregnancy to avoid nausea and gas. You should also consume enough water to help the fiber do its job. Constipation is a huge problem in pregnancy but stay away from laxatives and castor oil, the latter of which can prevent your body from absorbing the necessary nutrients.

Folic acid (man-made) Folate (natural) 600 micrograms daily	Decreases the risks of neural tube defects, such as spinal and brain abnormalities. Promotes blood and protein production. Enhances effective enzyme functions, which are crucial for cell division in your baby's development.

Folic acid can be taken as a supplement, but it can also be consumed naturally in food. It's hard to eat enough folate, so a supplement can boost your daily intake. Foods that contain folate are:

- Dark green leafy vegetables, asparagus, broccoli, Brussel sprouts, spinach, cauliflower, cabbage, leeks, parsley, and peas;
- Fortified cereals, bread, pasta, bran flakes, wheat germ, and whole-grain bread;
- Oranges, strawberries, fortified orange juice, tomatoes, and citrus fruits;
- Legumes, beans, chickpeas, unsalted peanuts, and walnuts.

Iodine 260 micrograms daily	Improves fetal brain and nervous system development. Produces the thyroid hormone for growth and development.

Iodine is necessary during pregnancy and breast-feeding, and it's found in eggs, dairy products, seafood, and seaweeds like nori and kelp.

Iron 27 milligrams daily if you're pregnant 10 milligrams daily if you're breastfeeding	Promotes hemoglobin, which is the main protein found in red blood cells. The red blood cells carry oxygen throughout the body. Prevents anemia, which is a shortage of red blood cells. Decreases the risk of infections. Improves energy levels. Ensures better organ function and development for you and your baby thanks to the increased oxygen circulation. Relieves depression and irritability.

Iron should be eaten with vitamin C for better absorption. Consuming too much iron can result in nausea, so don't overdo it. Iron is more easily absorbed through eating meats more than plants. Iron-rich sources include:

- Fortified breakfast cereals, enriched grain products, soft pretzels, fortified rice, and whole-grain bread;
- Lean beef, poultry, shrimp, sardines, salmon, tuna, lamb, and pork;
- Leafy green vegetables, broccoli, Brussel sprouts, collards, sweet potatoes, lima beans, turnips, and black-eyed peas;
- Dry beans, soybeans, peas, peanuts, pumpkin seeds, almonds, Brazil nuts, and lentils;
- Apricots, dried prunes, raisins, grapes, oranges, plums, watermelon, all berries, and grapefruit;

- Hard-boiled egg yolk.

Protein See the servings recommendations.	Promotes cell growth and blood production. Regulates fetal development, including the heart and brain. Reduces your anxiety.

Protein provides the building blocks for your baby to grow and develop healthily. Even vegetarians should be sourcing protein while they're pregnant. There are two kinds of proteins, namely animal-sourced and plant-based.

Animal-sourced protein includes:

- Seafood;
- Lean meat products;
- Poultry;
- Egg whites;
- Dairy products.

Plant-based proteins include:

- Quinoa;
- Tofu;
- Beans, lentils, nuts, seeds, nut butter, and legumes.

Vitamin B6 Speak to your doctor about your dosage.	Promotes red blood cell creation and health. Aids the effectiveness of protein and carbohydrate processing.

Vitamin B6 is found in pork, wholegrain cereals, and bananas.

Vitamin B12 Speak to your doctor about your dosage.	Promotes red blood cell health. Improves nervous system development for the baby.

Vitamin B12 is essential as a supplement for vegetarian moms-to-be. For non-vegetarians, it can be found naturally in poultry, seafood, meat, and dairy products.

Vitamin C 80 - 85 grams daily	Enhances dental health. Assists with iron absorption.

You can add vitamin C to your daily diet by including:

- Citrus fruits, fortified fruit juices, papaya, strawberries, and tomatoes;
- Broccoli, cauliflower, green peppers, and mustard greens.

Vitamin D 600 international units daily	Assists with calcium absorption. Boosts your immune system. Helps with your baby's development and growth.

Vitamin D is easily absorbed by spending time in the sun, but it can also be added to your diet. You may want to ask your physician to test your blood and let you know your current vitamin D levels. Many products containing calcium are also fortified with Vitamin D because the body requires it to absorb calcium. However, vitamin D is also found in fortified cereals, bread, and milk.

Food Groups and Sizes

Daily consumption of foods with the right nutrients helps you to sustain a healthy and happy pregnancy. The secret to nutrient-dense fruits is that they are much brighter in color. The more color you see, the more nutrients it holds. Any nutrients you feel can't be met through your diet should be discussed with your doctor, who can prescribe a prenatal vitamin. A prenatal vitamin can enrich your diet either way and is recommended for optimal nutrition.

There are five major food groups you should include in your diet to maintain a healthy pregnancy. The chart below will guide you on the recommended number of daily servings and the serving sizes of each food group.

Food group	Daily servings	Examples of serving sizes
Fruit	2	1 medium apple, orange, or banana. 2 small apricots, kiwis, or plums. 1 small cup of diced canned fruit without added sugar. 4 fluid ounces of fortified fruit juice. 30 grams of dried fruit (occasional treat)
Grains	8.5	1 slice of bread. ½ cup of cooked rice, pasta, barley, polenta, porridge, noodles, or quinoa. ¾ cup of wheat cereal flakes. ¼ cup of muesli. 3 crackers. 1 muffin or scone.
Lean meats and other proteins	3.5	2 ounces of lean beef, pork, lamb, or veal. 2.8 ounces of thoroughly cooked chicken or turkey. 3.5 ounces of well-cooked fish. 1 small can of fish. 2 large eggs. 1 cup of cooked or canned beans, lentils, split peas, or chickpeas. 6 ounces of tofu. 1 ounce of nuts or seeds.
Pasteurized and reduced-fat dairy products	2.5	8 fluid ounces of pasteurized, low-fat milk or buttermilk. 4 fluid ounces of evaporated milk. 8 fluid ounces of soy and rice drinks (it must contain 250 milligrams of calcium per glass). 1.4 ounces or 2 slices of cheese.
Vegetables	5	½ cup of cooked vegetables, beans, peas, or lentils. 1 cup of green or leafy raw vegetables. ½ cup of corn. 1 medium potato or another starchy vegetable. 1 medium tomato.

You've probably noticed that some tantalizing foods are missing from the charts. Fat and carbs also make up part of your diet. However, you should stick to complex carbohydrates that keep you fuller for longer, such as whole grains, vegetables, baked potatoes with the skin on, beans, peas, and fresh or dried fruit. You should stick to monounsaturated and omega-3 fats, such as olive, coconut, avocado, and peanut oil. Tuna and wild salmon are also good options, and you can get fat from nuts, nut butter, and pasteurized butter (not margarine). Keep your fat intake to 30% of your daily calorie consumption. Anything more will only store more fat in your body than you need.

Try to follow the recommended servings daily for each food group, but don't beat yourself up if you struggle. A simple way to ensure you get maximum nutrition is to include an item from each food group in every meal, and add two different food groups to each of your snacks. Carry water everywhere you go, and always keep nutrient-dense snacks nearby for those munchies. Meal planning weekly can also make this a lot easier for your pregnancy brain, which is often forgetful or impulsive when you are trying to stick to your guns. Remember, you are not dieting, which isn't advised during pregnancy. You're merely making changes that will benefit you and your baby.

Pregnancy Superfoods

Some foods are jam-packed with the nutrients you need, and this makes them pregnancy superfoods. Some hidden gems bring big benefits (Taylor & Wu, 2020).

Superfood	Benefits
Avocados	This creamy dream gives you vitamin B6, folate, and monounsaturated fat. It also keeps you fuller for longer.
DHA-enriched eggs	This low-calorie protein helps your baby's eyes and brain develop without adding too many pounds.
Iron-rich foods	Duck, beef, spinach, dried fruit, and soy can keep you on track to a healthy pregnancy. Make sure you're eating enough iron, or get a supplement.
Mangoes	Who doesn't love the bright yellow sweetness of mangoes? Mangoes offer more vitamin A, C, and potassium than salads do. Wow!
Nuts	Nuts are dynamite in small packages. They contain calcium, potassium, magnesium, zinc, vitamin E, selenium, and good fats. They also make great snack options if you add some fruit to the mix.
Oatmeal	One cup of oatmeal can give you a third of your daily magnesium requirements, and it packs a powerful fiber punch to combat constipation. It also contains iron and vitamin B vitamins.
Yogurt	You can't usually go wrong with yogurt, even in the first trimester when your stomach feels like it's spinning. Yogurt contains healthy bacteria that maintain your gut microbiome, which is the billions of bacteria that absorb and process nutrients for you and the baby. Stick to plain yogurt, and add honey or dried fruit to sweeten the deal.

Other amazing foods you should try to include are wild salmon, lentils, edamame, and quinoa. Snack options are abundant in nutrient-dense foods. You can keep nuts, dried fruit, cheese sticks, yogurt, pita/bread, canned fruit, and hard-boiled eggs handy for when the hunger monster comes to town, which happens multiple times daily when you're pregnant.

Foods to Avoid

Some foods do more harm than good, but knowing about them can help you reduce or remove them, even if you've been eating them until now. You couldn't take away what you weren't aware of, so don't be hard on yourself if you've already eaten some of these foods during your pregnancy.

Unpasteurized foods are the first group of foods you can remove. It includes milk, juice, and soft cheeses. You should also avoid pepperoni, cold cuts, deli meats, and hot dogs. Also, be sure to avoid uncooked sprouts and fish known to be high in mercury content. Mercury is an unwanted environmental issue, and that's how it gets into your food. It accumulates in the oceans and rivers from air pollution, which then turns into methylmercury. This is then absorbed by the larger fish, especially fish that eat other fish. A diet with less mercury will prevent any harm in the development of your baby (Ben-Joseph, 2018). Read the label on your canned tuna next time. If it contains light tuna, it's okay to eat it in moderation, but if it contains albacore or white tuna, it's better to throw it out. Other fish with high-mercury content are:

- Swordfish;
- Shark;
- King mackerel;
- Marlin;
- Tilefish;
- Orange roughy;
- Big-Eye tuna;
- Raw fish.

The reason you should avoid unpasteurized foods is that they sometimes contain small amounts of food-borne bacteria that may enter the placenta and harm your baby. Before panic sets in, registered nurse Rebecca Decker explains that the amounts of bacteria in listeriosis as one example are normally minimal, and infections are rare (Schnabolk, 2020). Listeriosis can lead to miscarriage, stillbirth, and premature labor in rare cases, but only one in every 120,000 women gets listeriosis during pregnancy, so your risk is very minimal (less than .0001%). However, avoiding the roots of potential infections can help you keep your baby's development on a healthy track. Once again, don't be worried if you've already eaten these foods, and don't beat yourself up for letting it slip once in a while.

Foods we avoid to keep our babies safely away from infection are:

- Unpasteurized milk, feta, brie, camembert, and blue-vein cheese;
- Deli meats, cold cuts, sushi, ham, sashimi, uncooked salmon, and premade salads bought from the deli;
- Unpasteurized pates and meat spreads;
- Food and pudding containing raw eggs like tiramisu and mousse;
- Any soft cheese ripened and aged with mold;
- Homemade mayonnaise;
- Raw clover, radish, and alfalfa sprouts;
- Unwashed vegetables and fruit;
- Any raw, rare, or undercooked meat;
- Smoked meat or fish;
- Undercooked seafood like clams, mussels, scallops, and oysters.

Some foods can also contain E-Coli, salmonella, and toxoplasma bacteria, all of which you want to avoid exposure to as much as possible. The placenta is penetrable by many bad bacteria, but there are some tricks to use at home that will reduce your risk of exposure. Many of the bacteria can be killed with heat, so everything you cook should be freshly made and read 165.2° Fahrenheit on a kitchen thermometer. If it's cooked well and eaten fresh, you shouldn't have a problem with bacterial infections. Bacteria also don't like clean surfaces and hands, so wash your hands with antibacterial soap and hot water before and after touching meat or seafood. Disinfect your kitchen surfaces and fridge regularly, and wash raw fruits and vegetables before storing them. Cook your meals thoroughly with fresh, clean, and pasteurized ingredients to stay safe.

Remember to keep your caffeine consumption to four ounces or less daily, and avoid alcohol and drugs altogether. Some things are best avoided rather than trying to taper down. There isn't enough evidence to prove that certain amounts of alcohol are safe during pregnancy, so it's better to not take the chance if you want a healthy baby who has a bright future ahead of them. Start planning your meals, and don't leave food frozen too long, either. This can also cause bacterial overgrowth. Only heat can kill bacteria. Start adding nutritional foods to your diet so that you and your baby can benefit in a way that's fully in your control.

3

STEP 3: IT'S TIME TO GET OFF YOUR FEET! THE HOLY GRAIL OF SLEEP

There's one fear most moms-to-be face in early pregnancy or when they plan to have a child. With bated breath, we await the day our babies will need to feed every two hours, and we dread the lost sleep that comes with most newborns. However, we soon realize that sleep becomes an issue long before our gorgeous bundles arrive. Pregnancy and sleep are not friends. Between the heartburn and the restless legs, we find ourselves sitting in the bathroom for the fifth time before the sun rises. And just as we lay our heads to rest once more, we're jerked awake by the loud grumble resonating through the room as the snoring starts, and we quickly realize we can't blame our partner anymore.

Irrespective, sleep is the third step to a healthy and worry-free pregnancy. And yes, it's possible.

Better Sleep, Improved Results

Sleep is the third step of your journey because getting adequate rest reduces the risk of many pregnancy fears, such as complications, miscarriage caused by excessive stress, and stillbirth among others. Sleep has a relationship with every part of you and your baby's well-being. It's not only a time of rest, but it also restores the body and mind for better functions. Short-term memories are transformed into long-term memories while you sleep, which is useful when you have pregnancy brain. Your blood vessels are also restoring themselves, which matters because they're under additional pressure to supply your baby with oxygen and nutrients. You may not be eating for two, but you're certainly providing blood and vital functions for two. Your immune system also restores itself during sleep, lessening the chance of infection, and your blood glucose levels stabilize. Two hormones are responsible for sleep cycles, namely melatonin, and serotonin, and both of them regulate your insulin levels, which controls your blood sugar.

Moms-to-be often blame their pregnancy hormones for their moods, behaviors, and decisions, which is true, but losing sleep can alter the balance of hormones within your brain and body, changing the way you feel and think. Pregnancy brain is a real thing, and lost sleep worsens it. Insomnia may even be a habit brought into pregnancy from before. It's the inability to stay asleep, fall asleep, or cycle through the various restoration stages by sleeping deeply. Sleep is further interrupted by heartburn, restless legs, cramps, discomfort, and regular bathroom visits. It's not a good idea to ignore the way sleep affects you during pregnancy, so you should learn what you can gain from kicking your feet up.

A recent paper published in *JAMA Psychiatry* examined the benefits of helping 208 moms-to-be reduce insomnia during pregnancy with cognitive behavioral therapy (Felder et al., 2020). The moms-to-be were taught how to sleep better with practical advice. Getting better sleep reduced anxiety, depression, fear, and stress among the participants. The moms-to-be were able to get the rest their bodies and minds needed.

Better sleep can also reduce potential complications during pregnancy (De Bellefonds & Rebarber,

2021). Improving your sleep quality is another way to prevent preeclampsia, gestational diabetes, stillbirth, preterm labor, and high blood pressure. Losing some sleep during pregnancy is normal and expected, but women who sleep seven hours or more at night can significantly reduce their risk of having a c-section. To put the icing on the cake, they can also shorten their labor because their bodies are better prepared after restorative sleep. Never underestimate the value of good sleep again, and follow the tips you are about to discover to give yourself the best chance of getting a great night's sleep.

Setting the Stage for Great Sleep

A few simple changes can set the stage for improved sleep. The first rule of setting the stage is that you should cut out everything that messes with your sleep hormones before bed. Avoid drinking or eating caffeine within two hours before you sleep. Keep in mind that chocolate also contains caffeine, and so do some teas. Don't exercise within two hours of bed, either. Exercise can energize you, which you'll learn more about in step four. Most importantly, get rid of screens one to two hours before you sleep. Screens emit blue light, which tricks the brain into believing it's daytime. Blue light can also alter your sleep cycle hormones, preventing you from switching off. Creating a relaxing bedtime routine is a way to encourage drowsiness. Make sure you're comfortable, too, even if you must own a mountain of pillows. Your pajamas, sheets, and room temperature should be sleep-conducive. Cool temperatures are often better during pregnancy.

Urinating frequently is one of the worst sleep disruptors, so set the stage by drinking most of your fluids early in the day. Only drink at night to quench your thirst, and nothing more. A small glass of warm milk is an option, but keep the majority of your water intake for during the day. Your kidneys are already working overtime by filtering the excess blood during pregnancy. You also have high levels of human chorionic gonadotropin (hCG) hormone, which makes you pee more. The third trimester will come with pressure on your bladder, so there's no way to stop the frequency of your bathroom visits without controlling when you drink fluids. Gain the right control over your fluid intake during the day, and you might just sleep through the night.

Be consistent with your bedtime, too. Ironically, you'll find out how valuable consistency is when your baby arrives. Consistent parenting is how you raise well-adjusted and successful children. Anyway, be consistent with the times you go to sleep and get up in the mornings. Treat yourself like a baby on a sleep schedule. Weekends should be the same, too. Resting during the day can help you catch up with some lost sleep as well. Naps are encouraged, as long as you don't sleep too long or too close to bedtime. Midday or early afternoon naps that last an hour are a good energizer to get you through to the end of the day. Once your stage is set for improved sleep, you can then focus on specific sleep problems common in pregnancy, and how to overcome them.

Common Sleep Issues

Some common sleep problems may occur during pregnancy. Seventy-eight percent of moms-to-be experience the conundrum of wanting to sleep but being unable to do so (De Bellefonds, 2019). The sleepless nights normally come in waves, and the waves are much like those in the oceans; they can't always be predicted. Admittedly, the waves of the oceans also resemble the bladder's need for relief during pregnancy. Every time you think it's over, another hurricane seems to hit the shore! Anyway, this won't be a problem after you properly set the stage for sleep.

Heartburn

Heartburn is experienced because pregnancy hormones relax the muscles that keep stomach fluids and acids inside the stomach. And of course, they relax these muscles more at night. Heartburn may surge to a more painful experience in the third trimester because your baby bump begins pushing up against your stomach. As cute as baby bumps are, they can also cause a little discomfort, but I promise, it's worth it when you meet your baby. Preventing the worst of heartburn is simple if you don't eat large meals within two hours before bedtime. A full stomach means more indigestion. You should also prop your head up higher with pillows. Your partner needs to know one thing; pregnant women require about 500 pillows! They'll get used to it. You can also take pregnancy-safe Tums, which is an antacid that contains calcium, and you should avoid foods that cause acidity later in the day. Stay away from spicy, greasy, and carbonated foods and drinks. Avoid chocolate, tomatoes, and citrus before bed, too.

Leg Cramps

Leg cramps are another daunting part of sleepless-ness in pregnancy. Your body's carrying extra weight, and this causes compression of the blood vessels. Leg cramps come at any time, although they're most common at night. Stretching your legs can improve blood flow and lessen cramping. The easiest one to do is to straighten your leg while gently bringing your foot toward you, without stressing your toes. Doing some stretches before bed can prevent the cramps so you don't find yourself rushing to the safety of an ice-cold floor, which also relieves the cramps a little, but it's not pleasant in the middle of the night. Leg cramps can also be a sign of dehydra-tion, meaning you should increase your water consumption during the day. Just remember not to increase it when a cramp strikes at midnight, or you'll be back in the bathroom a couple of hours later. A lack of magnesium and calcium also leads to leg cramps, so consider increasing your intake, or speak to your doctor about increasing it in your prenatal supplement.

Nasal Congestion and Snoring

Nasal congestion is another commonly-shared problem among moms-to-be because the hormones estrogen and progesterone increase your blood levels throughout your body. Blood flow to the nasal membranes also increases, which makes them produce more mucus. A stuffy nose may even become a post-nasal drip that causes a cough in later pregnancy. It's nothing to worry about, and you can use nasal strips to ease the congestion for a medicine-free solution.

Snoring may also result from congestion because the airflow through the excess nasal mucus becomes strained, making you breathe through your mouth. Be sure to mention snoring to your OB-GYN when you visit again because it can also be a sign of sleep apnea, which is momentary pauses in breathing. You may need to test your blood glucose or pressure to be sure you and your baby are doing just fine. However, chances are that congestion is causing the roof-raising snores from you during pregnancy. Your partner can purchase some earplugs if necessary.

Restless Leg Syndrome

Be aware of restless leg syndrome (RLS) as well. It's not the same as leg cramps. RLS is when your legs gain a mind of their own while you're sleeping. Suddenly, you feel this tingling as your legs gain an unexplainable urge to move. Moving them only relieves the restlessness for a few seconds before the urge builds again. RLS may indicate a shortage of iron, so speak to your doctor about testing your levels and adjusting your intake. Relaxation techniques, avoidance of stimulants before bed, and wrapping a warm cloth over your legs at night can also relieve RLS.

Making sure your bedroom is sleep-friendly and you have solutions to potential disruptors can reduce sleeplessness also.

Kicking it Down a Further Notch

Improving something normally requires us to kick it up a notch, but promoting deeper, more peaceful sleep means we should turn it down a little. There are four great ways you can promote your sleep quality and length to help you transform sleepless-ness into a dream—pun intended.

First, improving your bedtime routine with new tricks can help you sleep better. It's all about relaxing your mind and body for optimal downtime. You can take a warm bath for 20 or 30 minutes before falling asleep. Don't get into a hot bath because pregnant women are already hotter than normal, and it can affect the baby. Warm water can soothe your muscles, but hot water will overheat your core temperature. Body temperature before bed is important because it drops as you fall deeper into the sleep cycles. Lavender is a useful spray, oil, and lotion you can use to promote better sleep. I often recommend it to anyone who suffers from depression and anxiety. It calms the mind through your senses. Spray some lavender on your pillow, or ask your partner to rub some lotion into your skin.

Comfort is another way you can support better sleep. I won't forget my husband's face when he saw I had added even more pillows onto the bed one night. I could see the worry in his eyes because the poor man hardly had space left as it was, but he's a supportive person who conjured the willpower to not press my pregnant buttons. His facial expression said enough, and his calmness seemed so forced when he said: "Oh, you got a few more." Anyway, pregnancy pillows are specially designed for maximum comfort. The best way you can sleep, especially once your belly grows, is on your side. The left side is best because sleeping on your stomach automatically becomes impossible, and sleeping on your back isn't advised past the first trimester. Other than the snoring it may cause, the weight of your growing baby may press on the intestines and the vena cava, which is the main artery that brings blood back from the lower body.

Again, don't panic if you wake up in the wrong position. The fact that you wake up is a sign that your pregnant body decided you were lying wrong. It's natural to roll over during the night, but your belly will signal to the brain that you need to turn again, so don't let this worry you. Pregnancy pillows can help you enhance your comfort. A pregnancy wedge can be placed behind your back while you lay with a pillow between your knees. You can also get full-body pregnancy pillows that allow you to lie cradled in a suitable position or get c-shaped pillows that support your knees, belly, and back at the same time. Finally, you can increase your sleep sanctuary with relaxation techniques. Listening to calming music for 30 minutes, or practicing meditation or visualization before bed is proven to improve the quality and duration of your sleep (Miles & Mindell, 2020). That brings us to the three other techniques that promote improved sleep.

Deep breathing is the second activity you can use to improve sleep. Deep breathing is about using the most natural thing on earth—oxygen—to calm your mind and body enough to cause drowsiness. Deep breathing encourages you to draw air into the deepest parts of your body, which is either the diaphragm or core, both of which surround your baby. Lie on your side in bed if you have a big belly. Straighten your legs and take a deep breath through your nose. Allow the breath to flow as deeply as you can, and be conscious of how your belly moves forward. Hold the breath before you gently allow it to exit your nose again. Notice how your belly returns as the air passes out.

Guided imagery is the third activity you can use to promote quality sleep. You should make yourself comfortable and close your eyes before using your imagination to paint a calm and inviting mental picture. You want to imagine yourself in a place that makes you feel relaxed and peaceful. It may be in front of a fireplace where you can imagine focusing on the flames dancing back and forth. It may be on the warm sand on a beach where you can watch the clouds pass overhead, or it can be your favorite place in the woods. The secret to turning your imagined place into a calm and sleep-inducing picture is to use your senses to smell, taste, hear, see, and feel everything you can. Listen to the crackling flames of the fire, watch the shape of each cloud on the beach, and smell nature at its finest after it rained in the woods.

Progressive muscle relaxation (PMR) is the fourth activity you can use. Practicing PMR can help you feel in control of your body at a time when it feels impossible, which makes you feel more relaxed. Lie on your bed as you focus on your jaw and facial muscles. Try to tense them for a moment before releasing them. Pay attention to the changes in your physical sensations when you tense and release each muscle group as you move to your shoulders. Continue tensing and releasing muscles down your arms and into your hands before you move on to your thighs. Progress to your calves and then to your feet. If you don't feel relaxed enough, reverse through the muscle groups until you reach your face again.

Sleeplessness is history, and quality sleep is a gift for moms-to-be. Enjoy every moment of it because it will get harder when your bundle of joy arrives.

4

STEP 4: I LIKE TO MOVE IT, MOVE IT. EXERCISE EARNS A PRIZE

*A*nd the award goes to the pregnant mommy in the background dancing to the sound of animated lemurs! Exercise feels like the last thing you can accomplish once the pregnancy fatigue sets in and your back hurts under the weight of your belly, but it holds many rewards if you can implement it as early as possible. Moving your body is encouraged throughout pregnancy, and there are many ways you can do it safely. The fourth step on your journey is to create a healthy, happy, and worry-free pregnancy by moving your body.

Why Exercise Matters

Exercise is a gateway step to deal with many of the fears common in pregnancy. It can reduce the risks for gestational diabetes, preeclampsia, miscarriage, preterm labor, and birth defects. Exercise can also decrease worries about weight gain and whether you'll lose weight after your baby comes. You'll have better control over your emotions and reduce stress, anxiety, and depression. Moreover, exercise can help you manage labor better because you're strengthening the muscles you'll use during birth. Exercise is the foundation of improved health, so why would it be any different when you're pregnant? Remember that pregnancy is a blessing and not a disease. You aren't sick, and you can move your body to the rhythm of whatever feels comfortable for you.

It goes without saying that you should consult your OB-GYN before establishing an exercise routine. Every mom-to-be is unique, and your doctor has your medical records from before and during your pregnancy. They'll know what's best for you, but chances are, they'll motivate you to start exercising right away. Maintaining a regular exercise routine throughout pregnancy can help keep you and your baby healthy. Exercise can also keep gestational diabetes and preeclampsia away (Hecht, 2006). It boosts your mood, and it helps you sleep better. Exercise produces a biochemical reaction in the brain, releasing dopamine, serotonin, and endorphins, which act as mood elevators.

You can reduce stress and anxiety with exercise also. Moreover, the hormones adrenaline and cortisol, which are both related to stress, can be reduced as well. On a lighter note, you won't gain too much weight, and you'll find it easier to lose weight after delivery. Your energy levels will rise, which is just another benefit when you suffer from the fatigue common in pregnancy. Other advantages include reduced back pain and increased stamina while you're in labor. Who wouldn't want their endurance to increase during labor?

Using exercise can create resilience against the unwanted thoughts and behaviors that come with anxiety. Having a new perspective can allow you the clarity of mind to challenge thoughts and behaviors that hold you in a mental stasis. Your confidence will also grow, and you may even meet new friends among other expectant moms. Whether you were active before or not, exercise can only be good for you and your baby. It's best to ask advice from your doctor about how active you can be. Strenuous activity isn't necessary.

A brisk walk is suitable for exercise during pregnancy. You should be cautious about your chosen exercise routine if you have existing diabetes, heart disease, or asthma. You may not be able to exercise while you're spotting or have a low placenta or weak cervix. Once you have the go-ahead from your doctor, you can start planning your routine to enjoy the benefits of exercise during pregnancy.

The Plan

The universal recommendation for exercise during pregnancy is 150 minutes weekly, which is divided among five or more days. If you can manage to exercise every day, kudos to you. You will only benefit more from being active every day. The target is 30 minutes daily, but you can start with five minutes and work your way higher if you weren't active before becoming pregnant. The secret is to commit to regular increases if you start small. Ask yourself five questions and think about them before planning your exercise routine as a mom-to-be.

1. How often do I want to exercise?
2. What level of activity do I already accomplish?
3. What physical activities do I enjoy?
4. What stands in my way of being physically active?
5. Is there something that would encourage me to be more active?

The reason you should answer these questions is that you need to stick to your plan, and that can only be achieved if you have specific ideas, expectations, timeframes, and motivations. Choosing an activity that you enjoy can also make it easier to stick to your guns. One consideration you should remember when you plan your routine is that you'll probably have very little coordination and balance in later pregnancy, so keep that in mind while you choose exercises. Writing your plan out while you use the SMART goal system can also make it stick better, especially when you want to see your progress down the line. It also helps to keep your exercise plan written down to discuss it with your OB-GYN if changes are needed. The SMART system is a way to set goals.

- **Specific:** Outline precisely what and when you want to do something.

- **Measurable:** Highlight a timeline you can keep track of for rewards and progress. You won't know if you achieved your goal if you can't measure it.

- **Attainable:** This means you need to keep your pregnancy, moods, hormones, and energy in mind.

- **Relevant:** Indicates how this goal relates to your desired result. For example, aerobic exercises improve circulation, so they're relevant to pregnancy. Endurance training isn't as relevant.

- **Timebound:** This means you must choose a day and time to start your goal and end it.

If you want to write your exercise plans or cues in a chart, it may look like this:

Specific	Measurable	Attainable	Relevant	Timebound
Brisk walking	30 minutes	Mornings	Energy boost desired	Date (tomorrow)

This plan is simple. You want to walk briskly in the mornings, which is specific enough. You also want to do it for 30 minutes, which is measurable. You're choosing morning walks because you know your energy levels and time restraints, which makes your goal attainable. You aim to boost your energy, which is relevant, and you'll start tomorrow, which gives you a starting point. Be specific about the date though.

A few guidelines should be established before you go walking all over town.

- You want to wear light, breathable, and comfortable clothes. Indeed, this could be an excuse to go shopping, but you should also remember that pregnancy gives you an excuse to dress comfortably. Your metabolism is running at full steam, meaning you can overheat quickly, so stick to comfy and cool clothes.
- Wear shoes with a good supportive sole that won't hurt your feet. Once again, you have an excuse to look comfy, so own it. Your shoes must fit well, and there must be no

risk of falling or tripping. Tripping isn't funny when it's a pregnant woman.

- Schedule your exercise routine for the same time every day. Allow exercising to become a habit.

- Don't exercise within the two hours before bed, or you won't easily fall asleep.

- Warm-up with some stretches for five minutes before exercising.

- Drink water 30 minutes before and after exercise. It doesn't matter how many times you have to run to the bathroom. Hydration during workouts is not negotiable.

- Have a snack 30 minutes before and after working out. Bananas and fortified orange juice are great options because they contain loads of potassium.

- Reward yourself as you track your progress. The more you notice your progress, and the more rewards you enjoy, the higher your motivation climbs. Keep your rewards healthy like buying new baby clothes or getting a massage when you've completed a week's routine.

With a plan in hand, which was hopefully discussed with your doctor, you're ready to shake it up. We might not move like the lemurs in *Madagascar*, but we can certainly get groovy now.

Safe Exercises

Moms-to-be can safely exercise with low-impact exercises that don't require sudden movements or changes of direction. Flat and firm surfaces are best for you to prevent injuries, and you should always get up slowly to avoid dizziness. Make sure you're adding those 350 to 450 extra calories a day if you're physically active. Once you get into the rhythm of your workouts, the perfect exercise routine would start with five minutes of stretching, 15 minutes of cardiovascular exercise to get your circulation humming, and it would end with 10 minutes of a light workout. The uneven distribution of your weight will become a challenge for your center of gravity, so make sure you're using workouts that don't offset your balance.

Pregnancy hormones can also cause the ligaments to stretch between your joints, so the prevention of injuries is best achieved if you stick to low-impact movements. Avoid eating a large meal within an hour of exercising, too. A snack is advised, but a full stomach can make exercise uncomfortable. However, the most important rule for you to consider is that you should not exert yourself to a point of breathlessness. You should still be able to talk while exercising. It's not necessary that you can sing, but talking is a good way to know you aren't overexerted. A few popular options are safe for pregnant moms.

Abdominal exercises can help with back pain and poor posture when your baby gets heavier. The kneeling pelvic tilt abdominal is one such exercise. To do it, you get down on all fours, arch your back towards the ceiling, and gently tighten your abs while you hold the position. This helps to train your muscles for better posture when your belly grows. The standing pelvic tilt requires you to stand with your back against the wall. Your feet should be three inches out, and you'll tighten your stomach and buttocks while pressing your lower back gently against the wall. There are many other stretches that are beneficial during pregnancy, and a bit of research is all it takes to familiarize yourself with them.

Brisk walking is a favorite pregnancy workout. Walking allows you to elevate your mood and tone muscles while you're setting the pace. You can walk outdoors, or you can use a treadmill without an incline, although I would be very cautious if you choose to do so. Small inclines are encouraged as you progress in nature walks but don't ever set an incline on your treadmill. Sway your arms along your sides to get an upper body workout as well, and increase your distance weekly until you're enjoying 30 minutes daily. The beauty of brisk walking is that you can continue exercising as far into your pregnancy as comfortable.

Indoor cycling is great for amateurs and fitness fanatics. It allows you to boost your heart rate while you keep your joints safe and strong. Often the handlebars can be raised on stationary bikes, allowing you to adjust them when your belly expands.

Kegels are an expectant mother's best friend, and they can be done anywhere without anyone knowing. Kegels strengthen the muscles around the bladder, bowels, and uterus, making labor a lot easier when the time comes. Pretend that you're trying to stop a stream of urine by pulling the pelvic muscles tighter. Hold this for five seconds before you release, and then repeat it 20 times. You can do Kegels about five times daily.

Light weight training is a way you can tone up before and after birth. Make sure to lighten your workout if you were lifting weights before you became pregnant. Don't follow routines where you have to lie on your back. Also, don't start weight training if you weren't practicing strength training before pregnancy.

Low-impact aerobics or water aerobics boosts your feel-good hormones, tones your entire body, and works the heart and lungs to increase their fitness. Beginners should seek classes with a certified water aerobics teacher.

Swimming is a low-impact and weightless exercise, and no matter how big your belly grows, you'll feel like you can fly through the water. Swimming is a full-body workout that benefits you and the baby. It can also improve sleeplessness, reduce back pain, and relieve swollen ankles.

Exercises to Avoid

Anything that doesn't fall into the low-impact category should be avoided. Slow, smooth movements are best when exercising during pregnancy. There should be no bouncing, jerking, and *especially* twerking. Some things are better left unimagined. Comfort is another essential reminder during exercise. Heaving and sweating buckets aren't what you're aiming for. You and your doctor will know the best pace for you. Don't push it over the pace you feel comfortable with, and you can always switch to stretching and strength training when your belly grows too large. The weather can also make you overheat, so don't force yourself to complete an aerobic workout when it's hot and humid. Switch to stretching if the sun is beating down too hard.

Exercises you can happily avoid include:

- Activities where you can fall, such as horseback riding and skiing;
- Activities that encourage you to jump, skip, bounce, or run;
- Contact sports like basketball, softball, volleyball, and hockey;
- Deep knee bends;
- Double leg raises;
- Exercises where your belly can be jarred with movements or objects;
- Full sit-ups;
- Holding your breath while exercising;

- Straight leg toe touches;
- Waist twisting movements.

It's hard to imagine most of the exercises mentioned here being performed by a pregnant woman. Can you imagine a bunch of moms-to-be with huge bellies slamming into each other on the ice or sliding into home base? Anyway, the exercises in the list should also be avoided in early pregnancy, too. Your body has special requirements while you're growing a beautiful life inside of you. Treat your body with respect, and you'll see the results.

There are also signs you should stop exercising. Stop and call your doctor immediately if any of these signs are present:

- Abdominal, pelvic, or contraction-like pain;
- An irregular or rapid heart rate;
- A noticeable decrease in fetal movement;
- Chest pain;
- Difficulty walking;
- Dizziness, light-headedness, or faintness;
- Excessive nausea during a workout;
- Muscle weakness;
- Pain in your calves;

- Persistent headache;
- Shortness of breath;
- Swelling in your ankles, hands, calves, or face;
- Vaginal bleeding, a sudden downpour, or a steady stream of blood.

Being pregnant is a blissful time in your life, and no one knows your body better than you. Your instincts will tug at you if something's amiss, but you shouldn't be worried about exercising. Knowing the signs that you need medical care will ensure a safe routine, and you'll be working closely with your doctor before and during your workout plans anyway. You're more than capable of doing this because remember, pregnancy isn't a disease; it's a blessing.

5

STEP 5: STRETCH, REST, AND REPEAT!
PRENATAL YOGA ADDS TO THE QUOTA

*I*s stretching safe during pregnancy, or is the truth being stretched? Prenatal yoga wouldn't be so popular today if stretching was a problem. The keywords here are "prenatal yoga." Fortunately, pregnant women are treated specially in this world. You're special, and every technique is designed for optimal benefits because the world would be empty without moms. That's why an ancient technique like yoga was carefully designed to be both safe and beneficial when you attend classes specifically created for moms-to-be. The last thing we want is moms with big bellies burying their heads between their knees in the knee-to-ear pose. No, prenatal yoga is designed for your comfort and safety. It is one of the key steps to maintaining a stress-free and healthy pregnancy and can alleviate many of the worries in step one as well.

Special Benefits

Prenatal yoga can put one of the biggest fears to rest. It teaches you what to expect during labor, and gives you tools to reduce the pain. The fear of preterm labor can also be alleviated, knowing that yoga assists the body to maintain balance to potentially avoid early labor. Fears related to the labor process and expectations won't seem as frightening anymore once you become familiar with what can truly be expected. Best of all is that moms-to-be are taught stretches that can turn your worries into relaxed thoughts. Prenatal yoga is the essence of finding your balance and calmness while your mind prepares and calms itself for pregnancy and birth.

It's well-known in psychology that yoga, as well as meditation, are both beneficial to people who suffer from depression, anxiety, and chronic stress. An expectant mother's body is unusually stressed. Understandably, your body is both maintaining homeostasis while creating a new little being from scratch. Homeostasis is the body and brain's ultimate desire to maintain equilibrium and to see that nothing changes in your internal system. Pregnancy is obviously a change, so being pregnant and possessing primal instincts are like black and white. They're opposites, but opposites can also attract if a balance is found. You can establish the balance between the opposing sides, and prenatal yoga is designed to help you do just that. This might sound complicated, but all it really means is that while you are designed to try and avoid change to maintain your body's equilibrium, you can't avoid this change during pregnancy - which can lead to anxiety. Yoga helps your body and mind come to terms with the warring instincts inside you.

Promoting relaxation lets the body and mind know that everything's fine. There are no threats just because of a small change growing inside of you. The unknown is another major contributor to the stress response. That's why the common first-time pregnancy fears seem so daunting. It's hard for your mind to accept a new idea as something non-threatening. However, prenatal yoga introduces you to what can be expected, taking away the unknown factor. You start becoming more confident in yourself and your abilities. The right class will introduce you to breathing exercises, visualizations that take you into a labor scenario, and will have you practicing positions that may alleviate some of the labor pain naturally.

Your self-efficacy will also increase, which is the belief you have in yourself. You'll start believing that you can do this, and you'll hopefully hear from positive moms who've already been there. The University of Sao Paulo in Brazil conducted a first-hand study to determine how prenatal yoga affected pregnant women (De Campos et al., 2020). The women were interviewed at various stages of gestation to get a better picture of how they advanced with their yoga practice. The three key results seen in all the moms-to-be were improved self-knowledge, better self-care, and autonomy, which is self-belief. The Brazilian study showed that moms-to-be can gain a better sense of control over the situation, even during labor. The breathing and position practices strengthen pelvic muscles while they give women more confidence to do what needs to be done during labor.

This helps to reduce pain and discomfort for moms-to-be as well because a sense of control can trick the brain into believing that something isn't as bad as it was feared to be. The All India Institute of Medical Sciences also conducted a comprehensive review related to prenatal yoga (Mooventhan, 2019). A total of 53 studies were analyzed to make sure no stone was left unturned. The most phenomenal result among the studies was that prenatal yoga has vast benefits for labor. It reduced the time women were in active labor, and comfort levels for moms tended to increase before and after labor. The facts don't lie. Prenatal yoga is being studied thoroughly for a reason. There are so many more reviews, but I won't bore you with all the studies available. I'm merely sharing some incredible findings with you so that you understand how essential yoga can be on your journey.

You also don't have to be a seasoned monk to perform prenatal stretches. There will be no placing your legs behind your head, but prenatal yoga can teach you so much to make your entire journey as pleasant and exciting as it should be. Again, prenatal yoga is a combination of deep relaxation and preparation. Another study by the University of Worcester in England found out which prenatal yoga practices benefit pain reduction and confidence during labor (Campbell & Nolan, 2019). It turns out that positive influence during prenatal classes matters more than what you practice. Being surrounded by positive faces and instructors can further increase your confidence and reduce pain during labor. Positive affirmations taught in yoga classes also boost the chances of a better experience during labor.

Prenatal yoga is also a sleep aid for moms-to-be. Sleep problems during pregnancy don't only make the journey less exciting, they can also cause postpartum psychological issues, such as postpartum depression and anxiety. A lack of sleep can steal your mental well-being, but prenatal yoga is useful in restoring the body and mind to their preferred states. The fact that prenatal yoga puts your mind at ease and teaches you how to relax through poses and controlled breathing is the reason why you're able to fall asleep faster again. Some positions taught in yoga could be useful to improve your comfort at night, too. Prenatal yoga improves your quality and duration of sleep. Now, before you get bored into dreamland with science stuff, I want to share one more study with you.

According to a recent expert review published in the *American Journal of Obstetrics and Gynecology*, prenatal yoga can improve your overall immune system functions as well (Traylor et al., 2020). The review was a necessity when the pandemic hit. Everyone's stress levels rose, and that places a huge strain on the immune system. A hormone called corticosteroid can suppress the immune system when stress goes unchecked, and this leads to a higher risk of infections. If there's one thing you don't want, it's an increased number of infections during this happy time. A significant improvement in immune functions happened after only 20 weeks of yoga (Traylor et al., 2020). The moms-to-be averaged only two yoga classes per week.

Prenatal yoga can improve your journey on a whole new level. Learning more about your body and mind, and using this information to tune into the happenings inside of you can change the way your pregnancy thrives. You probably chose to be a mom not for the sake of fitting into the baby birthing trend among friends, but because you wanted to create life in its most beautiful form.

Take a moment to understand and accept the magnitude of this incredible achievement. Now, realize how much you want everything to go perfectly. Knowing your inner workings, and knowing how to change them can set the stage for an enlightened pregnancy. You want to remember every moment of this, and you desire the deepest connection to your baby. It starts by knowing what's happening and how you can make it even better. And if common worries still tug at your mind, remember that yoga also helps you maintain a healthier weight, especially in pregnancy. Prenatal yoga also ticks the self-nurturing box expectant mothers shouldn't forget. Moreover, it's an easy and fun way to grab the benefits of physical movement during pregnancy, even if you've never done it before.

That's what prenatal instructors and example-setting classmates are for, which brings the final benefit worthy of mentioning. Prenatal yoga classes allow you to build support groups and networks among other expectant mothers so you'll never be alone on this journey. Making friends with other moms-to-be can provide support, camaraderie, and the freedom to discuss fears with women who can honestly put your mind at ease. Besides, it's great to have friends with newborns when your baby arrives, too. At least you know they understand the mismatched socks and electrified hair when you arrive at their doors. They're familiar with the lost sleep that comes with a newborn, so there's no judgment. Rest assured, prenatal yoga is a winner, and it adds to the quota of what you and your baby need during pregnancy. And just when you think it can't get better, many of the reviews mentioned in this step have considered women with both difficult and regular pregnancies.

The only thing you have to do is check with your doctor or midwife, which should be done before any change in your lifestyle during pregnancy. Thanks to all the research done on prenatal yoga, chances are you'll get the green light.

What to Look For

There are countless types of yoga and instructors, and showing up at the wrong class with a pregnant belly will certainly earn you some odd glances. Some yoga instructors in regular classes are certified to teach pregnant women, but you have to mention it if you're not showing yet. The best type for you is prenatal or restorative yoga. Making sure it's a prenatal class will ensure optimal benefits for you and your baby. Qualified prenatal instructors will be up to date with research and techniques regarding pregnant women. They'll even know which asanas or poses are best for each trimester. Moreover, most allow you to try one class before signing up so you can see how nurturing and safe the environment is first.

Pregnant women have the benefit of using excuses other people can't, and being picky is another one you can gladly use. The vibe within the class matters. Remember the study that proved how positive vibes can promote better confidence and reduced pain? Look for a prenatal class where the atmosphere is positive and everyone speaks optimistically. Listen to the way the instructor and moms-to-be talk about pregnancy, labor, and expectations. You want people sharing the positive perception of labor and not the scary stuff. After all, you are bringing your baby into this world, and that's certainly exciting!

Surround yourself with moms-to-be who can lift your spirits and encourage your confidence to know that you can do this. Find a class where discussion times before or after class are prioritized. These are the classes where moms-to-be can share their experiences and learn from each other in a safe space. You don't want a class that's "wham, bam, thank you ma'am" with stretches alone. You want to talk and share. Some classes even bring new moms in to share their incredible experiences. You want positive stories and women showing off their gorgeous babies. This will also help you overcome the fear of the unknown.

What to Expect

First things first, your instructor should ask for some information about how far along you are, any discomforts you have, and what you're concerned about. This helps them cater to your individual needs with certain prenatal yoga practices. Your instructor will get to know you, and this helps because they might see you struggling with a certain aspect of your pregnancy journey, and may be able to help. They can pay special attention to helping you become more comfortable during positions you find challenging. You can also let your instructor know if there are specific body parts or positions, you'd like to focus on. You'll become familiar with bolster props in prenatal yoga, especially from the second trimester. Remember that you shouldn't lie flat on your back from the second trimester onwards, so there should be a bolster that elevates your upper body to offer support. The bolster can also be placed between your knees when you lie on your side.

The movements and stretches in this class will be gentler than regular yoga, and there will be a larger emphasis on your breathing. Some of the gentle flow movements may target your abdominal and pelvic muscles, and others might focus on opening your chest. Prenatal yoga also teaches you to breathe more deeply and evenly with diaphragmatic breathing, unlike Lamaze classes that focus on the short "hoo-hoo-hee-hee." Your instructor will gently guide you through stretching poses that relax your muscles deeply without you having to worry about over-stretching anything.

Stretching sessions will normally end with a savasana, which is a lying position for rest. Yoga promotes rest after stretches, and this is where the bolsters are most valuable. There are four main prenatal yoga practices you'll learn in class.

You'll practice various breathing techniques other than diaphragmatic breathing. We think breathing is natural, but we only realize how we learned to breathe when we're taught how to do it another way. You might use alternate nostril breathing, deep breathing, or mindful breathing, which makes you aware of your breath. Once you feel like you're in control of your breathing, you'll also feel more in control of the labor process and how you react to it. This way, you can make yourself feel calmer by simply applying controlled breathing.

You'll also practice mindful awareness of your body. Mindfulness suggests that we pay attention to sensations in our direct and internal environments in the present moment. Getting to know these sensations and learning to focus on them can familiarize you with your body, including your belly and your baby. You'll feel more confident and in control when you can mindfully pay attention to your body and movements, which increases your knowledge of how they work.

Another practice in prenatal yoga is to teach you about different positions, which helps you choose a better one during labor. The positions will feel odd at first, but that's okay. As the weirdness fades, you'll find yourself naturally entering a position that makes you feel more comfortable. You can't have too many tools when you get to the delivery room, and you'll be too engaged in your baby's arrival to worry about what people think when you change to an odd position. Indeed, by the time you are in labor, you will have practiced the different positions so often that they will be second nature, and you will feel much more in control.

The final technique you'll practice in prenatal yoga is modeled labor through visualization. What better way to familiarize yourself with the expectations of labor than to have a qualified instructor guide you through a visualization. It won't be scary if you choose the right class, so don't be worried about this.

And just like that, you take another step, or should I say a stretch into a healthy, happy, and safe pregnancy. Commit to just 20 minutes of yoga twice a week to improve your mood and dive into a better journey.

6

STEP 6: FEELING DISCONNECTED FROM THE JOURNEY? ANXIETY AND STRESS REDUCED FOR FINESSE

The nine steps you're learning are intended to aid you in having a joyful and healthy pregnancy, but stress and anxiety can be like barricades blocking your way. What would you do if barricades blocked the only route you had to get to the most scenic and wondrous part of a journey? Depending on the material of the barricades, it wouldn't be smart to plow through them unless you didn't mind a few dings on your car. However, mental barricades aren't made of concrete. They're made of intangible thoughts, fears, and emotions, which means with the right tools you can break through them. You'll notice them, but with every barricade you break through you will become stronger, and will be reminded of the beauty of the journey ahead. The sixth step in your pregnancy reshuffle is to learn how to smash the barricades and get back on the pregnancy journey so you can smile and anticipate the good stuff again.

The Truth

Anxiety and worry don't allow for a calm and collected pregnancy, and they keep you from focusing on the things you should (like the sweet baby growing inside you). Reducing stress and anxiety can decrease the risk factors for many complications because your body and mind can restore its resources to what matters—your gorgeous baby-to-be. You can reduce fears regarding labor, complications, the baby's well-being, and preterm labor. Lowering your stress levels reduces the risks for preterm labor, stillbirth, and underweight babies. Your fears are rooted in anxiety, and reducing it can even calm your nerves about breastfeeding after birth, bonding with your baby, and what kind of mother you'll be. The only priority is you and your baby right now. You don't need stress and anxiety taking away from how incredible this journey is supposed to be.

Instead of worrying about things you can't control, you should focus on the things that you can, one of which is the way you feel. Stress and worries only suck the joy out of pregnancy. You're not alone in your fears as you learned in step one. Anxiety and stress are present in 25 to 50% of moms-to-be (Traylor et al., 2020). The truth is that you need to decide if you want a pregnancy filled with happy and joyful moments, or do you prefer a worry-filled pregnancy? Our chosen perception of how we feel and react to situations can make a huge difference because it alters our decisions. Perspective is a delicate thing.

Do you want to create a deep connection with your baby and experience every moment of joy, or do you want to look back at this precious time with regret, wishing you'd been more present? Stress and anxiety are like common thieves that steal the joy from pregnancy and motherhood. Don't let this happen to you. Being free from anxiousness during pregnancy can bring benefits beyond joy. You'll have better concentration, your muscles will be more relaxed, and you won't feel irritable. Moreover, you'll sleep better, which means you'll store memories from this experience so you can hold dearly onto them when it matters most. You also won't have troubles with diarrhea, dizziness, restlessness, and shortness of breath, which are all common results of unchecked anxiety. Freedom from worry and stress in pregnancy can also reduce your risk of preeclampsia and preterm labor (Traylor et al., 2020). You can probably see how much more enjoyable your journey will be if you don't let worry take over.

Anxiety and stress place a strain on your body. Managing them prevents your baby from being seen as an unwanted change in your internal environment. You want your body to welcome the baby, and becoming the master of your emotions can help you do that. Understandably, there are numerous reasons to worry during pregnancy. Moms-to-be worry about their baby's health, or perhaps they stress about their own well-being. Worrying whether you'll be a good mother comes back often, but I'll say it again, worrying about it already shows that you're willing to do the best for your baby. If that doesn't make you a good mother, nothing will. Sometimes, being concerned about physical symptoms can also cause more stress than necessary. Stress is often the reason behind many negative symptoms, so worrying about it only makes it worse.

Feeling agitated, being unable to concentrate, and suffering from persistent digestive problems are just some of the ways stress can manifest. It won't help to stress about it further. It only helps to target your stress and fears to reduce them because that's within your control. The way you perceive stress is the key. Your expectations and speculations design your fears and responses. In most cases, speculations don't match the outcomes. Chances are that what you're speculating is actually much worse than reality, and that makes stress a daunting opponent. However, your perspective will change gradually once you learn how to manage stress differently. Now, you can learn to push back.

Daily Stress Reducers

Start sleeping between seven and eight hours every night. If you don't succeed tonight, try again tomorrow. Whatever you do, don't give up after having a bad night. Also, stick to your workout routines as they can reduce stress with feel-good hormones, and don't forget to sign up for prenatal yoga. Balancing your hormones with the nutrition you need while pregnant can soothe the emotional waves, too. Don't expect them to disappear entirely, and it's okay if you feel down or pressured today. It will happen, but try to aim for a better tomorrow. These are all wonderful daily habits to reduce stress and anxiety (as discussed in the previous steps), but there are a few more ways to make this journey blissful again.

Conscious Breathing

Breathing exercises are a valuable tool to practice, and you will learn some when you begin prenatal yoga. The key is to practice them daily, even when you feel great. With practice, you'll be in better control when you suddenly need them, and they will come more naturally to you. Spend 10 to 20 minutes daily breathing your stresses away. Sit in a comfortable position, like in a rocking chair or armchair. Close your eyes and imagine the issue that brings you worry or distress. Take a deep breath in as you focus on the issue while you count to five. Focus on how the air passes deep into your belly while it rises. Then, allow the air to press out gently as you visualize the issue streaming out of you with the breath you are exhaling. Repeat breathing in and out, and each time imagine the issue leaving your body. Once the tension is gone, focus on how relaxed your muscles feel. Picture yourself smiling as you continue to breathe evenly until calmness over-whelms you.

Thought Challenging

Challenging your thoughts can also reduce your fears and stress about pregnancy. Each time fear pops into your mind, take a moment to educate yourself about the facts behind it. Remember, speculation is almost always worse than reality! Create a worksheet for challenging your fears. Write each fear in your first column, and allocate a fact about it in the second column. Then, you can write down a way to reduce the fear or anxiety in the third column, and record the new way you feel in the last column. Complete a few rows until all your common worries are assigned to the worksheet. You can use more than one strategy and fact in the second and third columns. Keep this worksheet handy for daily visibility, and change it as new worries develop.

Fear	Fact	Strategy	How I feel now
Weight gain	25-25 lbs gained is healthy	Nutrition Exercise	Relieved/calm
Birth Defects	97% of babies are born completely healthy	Prenatal vitamin Dietary changes	Confident
I'm not a good mother	If I am worried, I am already starting to prioritize my baby	Nutrition Exercise Regular check-ups Bonding exercises with my unborn baby	I trust myself more

Self-Care

Daily me-time can also do wonders for anxiety and worry. You need time to yourself each day so you have the energy and resilience to better manage stress and anxiety when they do come. Making time for yourself may seem daunting when there's so much to do, but you have to prioritize moments to take care of yourself. Adjust the expectations of your responsibilities for the day so you have more time for yourself. Our expectations can often be unrealistic, especially during pregnancy. There's no such thing as a supermom. Well, at least not until she takes me time to recuperate and reenergize herself! Your me-time breaks don't need to be hours long, either. You can take 15 minutes to read a book, do a puzzle, enjoy some gardening, or go for a nature walk if you love being outdoors.

Try a new hobby during your downtime. You'll be surprised how much you can learn in nine months if you start knitting, playing an instrument, or writing short stories. You can also enjoy some adult coloring, and yes, it's both genuine and soothing. Paint a picture, learn a new language, or simply kick your feet back and watch a movie. Listen to some music or meditate. Call a good friend to chat about whatever makes you feel happy. Avoid conversations with negative undertones. Speak to people who raise your mood, and spend time with friends, having a light lunch or just a chat. Book massage therapy once in a while. It's deeply relaxing for moms-to-be. The possibilities are endless. The only reminder with me-time is that you must do what makes you feel better.

Making me-time possible is as simple as delegating chores and working less if you can. You're not turning the world on its axis, so it won't stop if you kick your feet up. Moms-to-be also tend to assume people know they need help. Everyone lives in their own bubbles, so don't expect friends and family to know what you need. Ask for help with chores and household responsibilities. Make a list of things people can help you with so the burden doesn't weigh you down.

Daily Journal Writing

Journaling daily is another stress-busting habit you should gain as a mom-to-be. It can also help you identify recurring triggers for worry and stress. Only once repetitive thoughts are identified can you determine how reasonable they are, and reframe them if they aren't helpful to you. Pregnancy journaling records your fears, emotions, experiences, and milestones. Your hormones are fluctuating, so you may not feel the same every day. Spend 15 minutes each night with your journal. Use your experience for the day as a prompt of what you should write, and however low you may feel at that moment, be sure to add one positive experience, thought, or feeling to your entry.

Mention how funny it was that you noticed how cinnamon makes you feel nauseous now but it was always your favorite spice. Write about your ultrasound and be descriptive about it. Write about how it made you feel when you heard your baby's heartbeat for the first time. Your pregnancy journals will be there as a reminder of how you felt in the precious moments, and this also helps when you need a little joyful boost when you read over them again. Journaling is also a healthy way to release emotions because stress is something we can't completely avoid. Journaling can help you restructure the way you see yourself and your pregnancy. You may identify repetitive thoughts while you validate your feelings.

Investing time in yourself daily to reduce anxiety and stress is encouraged in pregnancy. You don't need to keep yourself busy all day. You can take moments to invest in you and your baby's well-being throughout pregnancy. The more you invest, the larger your resilience grows, making worry about the things that rarely go wrong in pregnancy a manageable risk. Positive affirmations are another way to reduce stress daily, regain healthy thought patterns, and overcome unhealthy behaviors related to anxiety. We'll focus on them in step eight.

Long-Term Anxiety Crushers

Three long-term habits can reduce the power worry and stress hold over you. These habits require a little effort and time, but they help you regain confidence and resilience so you won't be overwhelmed by common fears anymore.

The first habit is that you should become a social creature with women in the same situation. Make friends with other moms-to-be and new moms so that you have a support network. Indeed, your partner, relatives, and current friends are there for you, but having friends who can relate is how you can share the burden of pregnancy worries. Remember to surround yourself with a positive group of women because negativity is contagious. Enlist a group of supporters who cheer you on and return the favor. Share happy and optimistic stories and hopes with each other. Every mom-to-be needs a support group to thrive.

The second habit is that you should readjust your expectations, and this also takes some practice. Think about where your expectations come from. Do they belong to you, or are they societal? Perfection doesn't exist, and if you're worried about being perfect, be assured that it's a societal expectation. Slowly let go of the expectations that you should be doing this, experiencing that, and feeling like a ray of sunshine every day. Unrealistic expectations can increase the weight of anxiety burdens. The truth is that you can't expect things to occur the same way they did for others. You can look at facts and statistics, and that way, you'll know what you're in control of changing and what can't be changed. Release the idea that you can control everything because you're holding yourself to unreasonably high expectations.

The third habit you should adopt is to practice relaxation techniques, such as guided imagery and visualization. Remember that you can control what happens in your mind if you use your senses to convince it to accept what you imagine. You can also use a simple mindfulness meditation where you sit quietly with your eyes closed and pay attention to your feelings. Mindfulness meditation is about remaining in the present moment as you remain aware of what you feel and think without judging yourself or your thoughts. Visualization involves imagining yourself in a place that brings peace while your eyes are closed. It could even be a fond memory. With all meditations, it's important to use your five senses to relax deeper. Guided imagery is another great option, and there are many apps that can help you while you learn how to meditate. Relaxation only gets better with practice.

Place your hand over your stomach for a moment, and close your eyes. Imagine your baby growing inside of you. Look at his/her little toes and fingers, and imagine listening to the heartbeat. Whenever you feel overwhelming stress or worry, just close your eyes and imagine watching your baby from inside.

7

STEP 7: I FELT A KICK! BONDING TO
AVOID DESPONDING

*W*e have this idea that our babies are only arriving when we enter the delivery room. Among the contractions and the inadvertent bone-crunching of our beloved partner's hands, there's also a sense of excitement and eagerness to meet this amazing human who's been growing in our bellies for nine months. This is where it becomes fuzzy because your baby has already been living inside of you, so the day of his/her arrival is not the day you're raising the roof in the delivery room. They arrived the moment an egg implanted itself in your uterus. Your baby became part of your life as soon as the seed blossomed into a heartbeat. Ignoring the developing baby during pregnancy means you have to catch up with the bonding you could have done from day one. Step seven is about bonding on a level that allows you to know and cherish the baby even before they arrive in the outside world.

Prenatal Bonding

Every mom and dad are eager to meet their little ones. Even though some fears may linger, the truth is that you're anticipating your baby's arrival as though your entire life is about to change, and it is. Bonding with your baby during pregnancy can decrease the fear of not being a good mother. It can reduce the fear of birth defects and developmental challenges. It can calm the waves of anxiety that may contribute to numerous risks. Bonding with the tiny human inside your belly can even make you see labor as less of an obstacle and more of a transition to meeting your new baby. What happens when you're overly excited about something? Time seems to move faster, and who wouldn't want labor to be perceived as shorter? Breastfeeding fears can also be tamed with prenatal bonding because you and your baby will already feel attached by the time they are born.

When you bond with your unborn baby, you become increasingly connected with your pregnancy, turning it into a positive experience. This bonding is highly beneficial to your baby, too. They can more easily connect with you after birth. The more connected you are to your baby before birth, the more positive your interactions with your newborn will be. Having this closer connection to your newborn will also help you navigate any worries you may have about doing the best for your baby. Developing babies already have intuition and emotional capabilities. They can feel what you feel. According to Dr. Carista Luminare-Rosen, babies can completely feel how much their mothers and fathers love them while they're still in the womb (Sorgen, n.d.). This allows them to know that the world is safe before they're even born. A baby who feels safe is much easier to parent.

Your baby can already gain trust in you and your husband, making your first parenting journey more enjoyable. Frequently talking to your baby in your belly allows them to recognize you and feel safe. You can't speak to them too much, and no one will think you're weird for talking to your baby belly in the middle of a mall. Ah, the things a pregnant woman can get away with! The fact is that while your baby is part of you during pregnancy, they're also individual beings with their own feelings, thoughts, intuitions, and emotional needs. You're achieving what's called parental reflective function once you consider your baby as a separate little being, and this creates a secure attachment for the baby. Bringing a securely attached baby into this world is what you want.

Secure attachment results in improved emotional, behavioral, cognitive, and social development, which also benefits your child in later life (Wheatley, 2018). A child's independence and confidence are partly grounded in having secure relationships with their parents, which starts before birth. The more secure a person feels, the more confident they feel in their own abilities. Bonding with your baby during pregnancy also has vast benefits on their prenatal development. Babies don't start learning language and listening skills after birth. Their hearing starts developing during pregnancy, and so do many other skills. Your baby is completely aware of your voice, emotions, and behaviors. They're listening and responding to all that you do. Research suggests that babies respond to their mother's voices, and they even remember songs they heard while in the womb (Apta Club, 2019).

Two studies were reviewed, and one showed that a baby's heart rate decreases while their mother speaks (Apta Club, 2019). The other study showed how a baby's movements slow down when they listen to their mother's voice. They actually pause their movements to listen to mama! Babies are most responsive to their mother's voice above all others, and they remember it after they're born. Calling them by their names or nicknames before birth can familiarize them with the sound of your voice, and this can help you have a soothing effect on them after birth. Your voice already starts shaping their understanding of the world in the third trimester. A baby's memory, social, and language skills are developing inside your belly, so talking to them, and visualizing your connection to them can create a shared experience. Unborn babies are aware of most of what's going on outside of mom's belly according to Michael Orlans at the Evergreen Psychotherapy Center (Orlans, 2015).

The awareness starts around 18 weeks when unborn babies start hearing the sounds inside your body. They can hear your heartbeat and the rumbles inside your stomach when cravings hit. An 18-week unborn baby can even rock themselves to sleep in your womb while you move, which can help you put a fussy newborn to sleep faster when you use a cradling motion to mimic the womb. From 26 weeks, your baby starts responding to noises outside of your body, and they may even be startled by loud or sudden noises. Their developing ears are sensitive. The 26-week mark is also when your developing baby can respond to the sense of touch. If you massage, rub, or gently press against your belly, your baby may respond. At 32 weeks, your baby starts recognizing vowels as their language development begins. This is why it's so important to speak to your bump in the third trimester.

Familiarize your baby with your voice, and let your co-parent do the same. It makes those sleepless nights a lot easier to manage once the baby's born if you can verbally soothe them. What you and your partner need to realize is that your baby is actively participating in conversations, workouts, and emotional changes within your body. They're not simply floating about, waiting for the day they enter this world. Your baby's senses and brain develop-ment are on track from early gestation, and you can control what influences the development of their future skills. Your baby is an individual with their own needs and transitions, but they're also sharing every experience with you and your partner if they get involved in the bonding exercises. Your attitude toward your baby is essential for their healthy development, so ignoring them won't bring an emotionally stable child into this world.

Recognize that they're waiting for you to speak to them. They're waiting to feel your touch, and they're waiting for their other parent to sing a weird song they made up. Babies love attention, so give it to them. And if there was any better news, it would be that prenatal bonding helps to prepare you and your partner for parenting. The Center for Family Research also reviewed 14 studies to further understand the positive outcome of prenatal bonding (University of Cambridge, 2018). One of the most important results found among the studies reviewed was that moms-to-be with an increased conscious awareness of their unborn babies led healthier pregnancy journeys. If you have any fears of being a bad mother, rest assured that being aware of your baby's needs in the womb will automatically make your maternal instincts kick into a higher gear. You'll feel motivated to lead a healthier and pregnancy-safe life until your baby comes along.

Prenatal bonding does so much for you as a worried first-time mom. It helps you see your baby as a real person. You feel more deeply connected to your baby and what's going on in your body during pregnancy. You'll also fast-track your attachment to this incredible bundle of joy once they're born. Being aware of your baby during pregnancy can also help you practice putting your baby's needs and feelings ahead of your own before they arrive. This makes you a great mother, never mind a good one. Ultimately, your fears about pregnancy and motherhood will decrease, and you'll start enjoying every moment of pregnancy, even when your baby kicks you awake at night. Allow your excitement about motherhood to grow while you're in the mom-to-be stage.

Ways Mom Can Bond

Pregnancy can be daunting for new moms-to-be, and the concerns often mask the excitement. The fact that we fear means we already feel attached to the baby. We're concerned about the well-being of this amazing child growing inside of us. And I'm no stranger to worrying about my baby during pregnancy. With my first child, I was initially a fretful mess – due in part to the fact that it had taken me 7 years and fertility treatments to even get pregnant. I worried about many of the common concerns discussed in step one, but because I had an understanding of psychology, I knew my fear could make me despondent if I allowed it to control my pregnancy. I came to the realization that I needed to take control of my pregnancy and my thoughts surrounding it. And so my journey to conquer my worries began. One of the first things I discovered was that a feeling of connectedness to my baby and my pregnancy was vital to relaxing and enjoying the experience. Prenatal bonding amplified my love for my baby and excitement for the journey, and it can do the same for you. There are numerous ways you can bond with your baby.

Have conversations with your baby. Talk to them about positive things like your hopes, dreams, and how much you love them. Call them by their nickname or name if you and your partner have chosen it. It's a good idea to personalize your journey by picking names early. Naming the baby in pregnancy reminds you that they're individual little munchkins.

Many parents name their babies after birth, but they miss an opportunity to familiarize their babies with their names beforehand, which helps the baby respond better when you try to soothe them. The human voice is not distorted by the uterus, so speak to your baby and call their name, knowing they'll hear you. If you aren't comfortable naming the baby until you see him/her, that's okay too. In fact, both of my children were nameless until they were 5 days old! We are in the minority who like to see what name suits the baby after they are born. However, both children had nicknames from the moment I knew I was pregnant, and this is what we called them most of the time even after they were born. In this way, we were still able to familiarize them with their "name" and they responded to the nickname when it was spoken to them.

Talk to other people about your hopes and dreams for your baby, too. Tell them whether you think they'll look like you or your partner. Don't complain about pregnancy issues if you have an aching back. Focus on the happy things.

Singing to your baby can also soothe them, and you can repeat the same lullaby every night. This helps you put them to sleep once they're born, as they'll already know the melody and find it relaxing and soothing.

Play music for your baby, but remember the startle response. Don't play music too loud, and don't put headphones on your belly. This could harm the baby's hearing. The best kind of music to play for an unborn baby is classical or any music with a beat that matches your heart's rhythm. Low-frequency sounds also penetrate the womb better.

Have an ultrasound done, and invite your partner along. The newer 3D scans really help you see every detail about your baby, and you can talk to your baby as you watch them on the screen.

Wait for your baby to kick and then gently press back on your belly where you felt it. The baby may love this attention and return the embrace. You can also encourage the baby to move and kick by massaging your belly. You should only massage your belly in the second and third trimesters, however. Avoid massaging your belly before this. You can also improve the experience by using lavender, frankincense, ylang-ylang, or olive oils. These oils are well-known for relaxation. Moreover, these oils can soften your belly, and they work wonders for mild pains during pregnancy. Giving your unborn baby a massage relaxes both of you.

To increase your connection with your baby and journey, you can also plant a tree in the backyard. This tree will grow with your child, and it allows you to nurture something representing your unborn baby. Don't forget to keep nurturing it when your baby's born, and get your child involved with the tree when they're old enough. Otherwise, you can also increase your excitement about your baby's arrival by hand-making items for him/her. Knit booties, paint, draw, and cross-stitch items for your baby. Booties are so darn cute, and they tend to create an 'awe' moment.

Create a time capsule for your baby, which helps you feel closer to them, and it's a wonderful gift for them when they're older. You can add a hand-written letter to your baby. Write to them about your dreams, hopes, and deepest desires for their future. Tell them how excited you are to meet them one day, and share your imagined ideas of what they'll be like. You can also add a pregnancy journal to your time capsule. Create entries of your experience daily, and be emotionally descriptive about your milestones as you reach them. A pregnancy journal helps you focus on your baby and the pregnancy, but it also allows your child to one day read a diary of their unborn life.

Finally, add a pregnancy scrapbook to the time capsule. Add ultrasound photos, colorful decorations, and fun news articles. Add pictures of yourself having a pregnancy photo shoot once a month. Children love seeing how their moms expanded during pregnancy. Take photos of your partner cuddling your big belly, and add many visual pages to your journey. This excites you and brings you closer to your baby, and can you imagine handing this time capsule to your child one day?

Go for mindful walks as you imagine your baby rocking to sleep in your stomach with each step you take. Touch your stomach, and allow yourself to feel deeply connected to your baby.

Behind your closed eyes, meditate with your hands on your belly as you imagine your baby inside you. Visualize them sucking their thumb, rolling around, and kicking. It's fun to see if your baby looks anything like you imagined once they are born.

Ways Dad Can Bond

Dads have a small disadvantage while expecting a baby. They can't feel the baby moving in their bellies, and they may feel like outsiders on this journey. However, they can still bond with their unborn babies, it usually just takes a little longer. With a little effort from dad, which is encouraged, he can also connect with his baby. Dads will also benefit from this when their babies learn to recognize their voices. There are a few ways dad can bond with his baby.

Dads can start with belly massages while mom kicks her feet up a bit. Your baby may respond to your touch as well if you place your hands on your partner's belly. Try to guess what you feel when movements occur. Perhaps it's a kick, or maybe you're feeling the baby's knees. Even just this little guessing game will make dad feel closer to the baby. It draws baby into your conscious thoughts and encourages you to visualize them. Just remember to be gentle when you massage mom's belly in the second and third trimesters.

Rather than waiting to hear from your pregnant partner while you're at the office, attend ultrasounds, birthing classes, and doctor's appointments with her. There's a huge difference between a blob on an ultrasound photo and actually being present while the baby moves around. You can't compare a photo to a movie, can you? A fun way to bond is to photoshop the ultrasound picture. Add some color and funny baby accessories, and upload it to your social media pages. This adds a little fun and humor to the journey, both of which increase your attachment further.

Take maternity photos monthly, and make sure you're a part of them. Then, stick them up on a special Facebook page created for your baby. Obviously, they won't be using the page for years, but this helps you store the journey of their earliest days in the cloud.

You should also be conversing with your unborn baby. Talk to the belly, and sing your baby a song. It works even better if you make the song up yourself because this personalizes your attachment to the baby even more. It makes the baby more real, and the additional effort increases your attachment. You can also read the baby a story every night to start a bedtime routine. Choose books you loved as a child to strengthen the bond. Make a playlist of music you'd like your baby to listen to, which encourages you to think about their emotional needs. Just remember to use positive and non-startling songs.

Be involved in purchasing furniture, clothes, and supplies for the baby. Dads should try to be involved in pregnancy and hospital planning as well. Be part of decisions, and think of something you want to do with the baby when they arrive. Perhaps you want to teach them to play catch, so buy a baseball mitt. You can also buy your favorite team's jersey in infant size, and it doesn't matter if you're having a girl or boy. Girls love sports too.

Don't feel guilty if either of you can't bond at first, because it is difficult before the baby arrives. Just keep trying, and the bonding will come when the baby's born for sure.

8

STEP 8: THINKING YOUR WAY TO A WORRY-FREE PREGNANCY - LET'S PRESCRIBE A POSITIVE VIBE

*H*ave you ever seen someone talking to themselves, and you don't see a phone in their hands? Perhaps they know the secret of using positive affirmations to convince their brain to believe what they are saying. No, they're not crazy. In fact, they might be on their way to a job interview and they're building confidence. Moms-to-be can also use optimistic thinking when doubts and fears creep up. Having a positive mindset helps you focus on the things that make an actual difference in your pregnancy, and it's the eighth step of creating a worry-free pregnancy.

The Power of Optimism

The key advantage of having a positive mindset is that you can gain control of making your pregnancy the best it can be, much like you do with your nutrition, exercise, sleep, bonding, and feelings. Most of what you worry about can be controlled and reduced if you change your perspective. There will always be things we can't control, but the steps in this book give you the power to regain control over what **can** be controlled. You can reduce your fear of morning sickness, weight gain, and what maintains your baby's growth and development with exercise and nutrition. You can decrease the risks of pregnancy complications, birth defects, and preterm labor by shifting yourself into a mindset that motivates you to control your lifestyle during pregnancy. You won't fear labor as much when you understand it more, and your mindset can help you adopt the changes you need to reduce the fear of the unknown.

Adopting optimism helps you overcome your worries about breastfeeding and being a bad mother. You can control your stress and anxiety with a different set of beliefs, especially believing that you can control certain benefits and risk factors. Your thoughts will control the way you behave, and how much you enjoy your pregnancy journey. You can either be the nervous woman sweating through her snow-white shirt on the way to her interview, or you can be the random woman saying affirmations to herself who gets the job. Your thoughts, beliefs, and actions are within your control, and that's what makes optimism such a powerful tool. Positive thoughts lead to positive feelings and actions.

Reframing negative thoughts into positive ones is possible, and it costs nothing. Psychology tells us that thoughts that are based on our beliefs will alter our feelings, which can then manifest as physical symptoms. The physical symptoms can then impact our behavior and decision-making, and this leads to more feelings of doubt, fear, and anxiety, which ultimately circles back to create a thought again. It's a cycle that happens within split seconds.

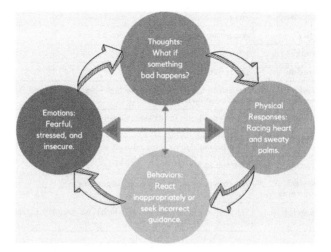

With time, thinking patterns are created within your brain. It's habit to start thinking a certain way. That's why people naturally lean toward either negativity or positivity. Every time you're experiencing something during pregnancy, a thought pops into your mind, and this is what it might look like if you're negative:

Experience	You watch a movie in which a woman has a c-section.
Belief	Women are bedridden for weeks after a c-section.
Thought	What if I need a c-section?
Emotion	You're frightened.
Physical symptoms	Racing heart, sweating, dizziness, high blood pressure, and the stress response is activated.
Behavior	You call the doctor to talk about c-sections.
Thought	The doctor asks to see you. (Which might be to calm your nerves, but reasoning doesn't come naturally here.)
Emotion	Your fear increases.
Physical symptoms	Weakness, nausea, and increased palpitations.
Behavior	You start consulting the internet, which is not generally a great idea, and really freak yourself out.

This is what a negative thinking pattern looks like. Now, change this to someone with a positive mindset.

Experience	You watch a movie in which a woman has a c-section.
Belief	Vaginal birth is best, but c-sections can be life-saving for baby or mother.
Thought	My plan is to give birth vaginally, but if a c-section becomes necessary I will do what is best for the baby and myself.
Physical symptoms	You are calm and relaxed.
Emotion	You feel confident that you will make the best decision if your birth plan needs to change.
Behavior	You imagine holding your baby after she's born, and already feel the love you will have for her.

There's a huge difference, and the mom-to-be who thinks positively, or at least chooses to do so, is the one who makes changes to what she can control. The way she thinks about the experience based on her beliefs is also referred to as her self-talk. She tells herself how she should perceive the movie. Mom one perceives the movie as something to fear, but mom two perceives it as a reminder that sometimes things change, and you must adapt. Your thoughts change the way you make decisions, and your self-beliefs impact your thoughts. If you're surrounded by negative people who amplify negative fears and thoughts, you'll more likely lean toward unhelpful behavior and negative self-talk. Keep this in mind with your friends and relatives. Negative thought patterns can also be called cognitive distortions. The most common anxious thinking patterns are seen below.

Conclusion jumping	You predict the worst-case scenario without facts.
Mind reading	You think your doctor is speaking symbolically, and you can read his mind under the hints.
Catastrophizing	You think small problems are huge. For example, you're so afraid of gestational diabetes that you think it would be the end of the world to have it (when really, those who get gestational diabetes only have to watch their diets more carefully, and the baby is not impacted much besides being a bit larger).
Emotional reasoning	You think things are worse than they are because you feel strongly about them.
Black and white thinking	There's no middle ground. Things will either go well or badly. This isn't a good way to think when you're pregnant because there are ups and downs, especially in your moods.
Labeling	For example, you keep telling yourself that you'll be a bad mom, even if there's no evidence.
Negative filtering	Your attention is aimed at the negative things instead of enjoying the precious moments, of which there are plenty.
Perfectionism	Yes, perfectionism is a distorted way of thinking because no mother or person is perfect.

These thinking patterns can change your self-talk and remove the joy from your journey. Healthy and positive thinking means you consider all the facts before deciding anything. You can do this by reframing the way you think. This thought reframing worksheet can help you do that.

Experience	You have a doctor's appointment.
Negative thought	Something will be wrong with the baby.
Emotion	You feel anxious.
Supportive fact	You ate something wrong yesterday.
Opposing fact	Eating a bad thing once almost never causes problems.
Challenging positive thought	The doctor knows what he's doing, and he can advise me on how to better curb my cravings.
New emotion	I feel calm and excited to see my baby.

Create a thought reframing worksheet for yourself, and continue practicing this exercise. The truth is that thinking patterns are often designed over years. They're habits, and habits don't change overnight. Give yourself time to slowly change your habits, and you can do this by practicing frequently.

Positive Affirmations

Self-talk is the way we think and talk to ourselves each and every day. It can either be positive, or it can be negative. Positive affirmations can be used to challenge or get rid of negative self-talk and must be practiced frequently to be effective. It may feel awkward or strange to talk to yourself at first, but with daily practice, you can change your thinking patterns. Over time, your new thought patterns will instill new beliefs. Training yourself to do this is important because people tend to be negatively biased, seeing the negative side before the positive one. Choosing to think positively will slowly help you move to optimistic self-talk with practice. Change your inner narrative about yourself with positive affirmations, and you can change your whole viewpoint.

A study published in *Social Cognitive and Affective Neuroscience* examined the changes in the brain when people practiced self-affirmations (Cascio et al., 2015). Functional magnetic resonance imaging (fMRI) was used to scan the brains of people practicing positive affirmations, and they found physical changes in the neural pathways in the brain. The prefrontal cortex was altered, and this is the source of reasoning. The self-value region in the ventral striatum also showed remarkable changes, meaning practitioners were valuing themselves and their abilities more. Self-affirmations can actually rewire your brain, change the way you think, and alter your self-beliefs. What can this do for moms-to-be? It can reduce stress and anxiety while eradicating doubts and fears. Positive thoughts are also followed by positive emotions, meaning you'll enjoy your journey again. Your confidence will grow as you become increasingly more present in your pregnancy journey.

Moreover, you'll have more strength to face any potential challenges during pregnancy. You regain the power you may think you've lost, and you'll be in better control over what can be changed. Ultimately, you'll have a different outlook on your pregnancy, and that will bring loads of joy back into this precious journey. You don't have to utter your affirmations in the elevator mirror in front of strangers. You can design affirmations at home, and repeat them daily in front of your own mirror, or say them silently in your mind. Standing in front of a mirror adds more emphasis to what you say, so you might want to give it a try. To create your own affirmations, begin by writing down your negative thoughts on paper. You can use the thought reframing worksheet to identify common negative thoughts that run through your mind. Once you have identified the pesky negative thought, create a positive one that challenges it. This is an ongoing exercise because new negative thoughts will pop up as the pregnancy progresses.

The worksheet also gives you insight into when the thought is triggered. You'll see which experiences may trigger unhelpful thoughts, and then you can make alternative thoughts visible by sticking notes in the right places. If you find yourself thinking negatively about breastfeeding when you see the milk carton in the fridge, then stick a note with your alternative thought on the fridge door. Stick notes in your car, on your mirror, and in your office. You want to challenge the negative thought as soon as it pops up, and you can do this by having reminders everywhere. Design a chart with the more common thoughts you want to challenge, and repeat these affirmations to yourself every morning and night. Repeating them about five to seven times daily is the best method to change a habit.

You can also use cue cards to write the negative thought on one side and the positive challenging thought on the other. The way you write affirmations makes a difference. Keep it simple with one sentence each. Don't use negative words like 'can't' and 'won't.' Negative words will only bring to mind the thought you're trying to change. You want positive images in your mind when you're reading them. For example, don't write: "I won't be a bad mother" which brings the thought of being a bad mother to the front of your mind. Rather write: "I'll do my best to be a great mother." When written positively like this, it brings the thought that you'll be a great mother to the forefront, and that's what you want. Don't write: "My baby won't have birth defects" which just brings birth defects to mind, but rather write: "My baby will be born healthy." Also, try to write in the present tense as much as possible. This makes it more real. To summarize your self-affirmation writing, you should:

1. Identify the worrying thought and write it on a chart.
2. Challenge the thought by asking yourself if it seems logical, helpful, or if you have control over it. Write down evidence to support and oppose your thought if there is any.
3. Replace the negative thought with your positive alternative.

4. Keep practicing your affirmations until they become a habit. They will become habits!

Specific Inspiration

Writing your own affirmations is the best way to change your self-talk, but sometimes, you might need inspiration. These affirmations are written for specific pregnancy fears, and they may help you until you write yours. Each fear also has a visualization prompt.

Breastfeeding fears can be soothed when you visualize yourself breastfeeding your baby contentedly while repeating a positive affirmation. Choose one of these affirmations to repeat daily:

- My body is designed for breastfeeding.
- My breast milk will be abundant, and it will nourish my baby.
- I trust my body, and I'll be able to feed my baby.
- My body is amazing and equipped to care for my baby.
- I'm prepared to learn how to breastfeed so my baby bonds well.

Labor fears can be reduced with a visualization of the process. Imagine yourself as realistically as possible in your birthing space. Include your support people or partner in your visualization. Affirmations for labor fears can include:

- My delivery will be healthy and beautiful, and I'm absolutely excited to meet my baby.
- My delivery will be wonderful, even if it doesn't go exactly as I plan.
- I'm one step closer to seeing my baby for the first time with every contraction I feel.
- The time for me to meet my gorgeous baby is closer with every push.
- My body knows how to give birth to my baby, and I'm the only one who can do this for my child.
- My body is ready to give birth, and I'm ready to meet my baby.
- I'm excited to my core to meet my bundle of joy.
- My body is wise, and it knows what to do.
- I look forward to a calm and peaceful birth.
- I trust that I can naturally give birth to my baby.

- I'll feel the closeness of my baby as the time nears.
- I have faith that I can tolerate any pain to see my baby's face.

Being worried about your ability to be the best mom can be soothed with a visualization about what type of mom you want to be. Write little sticky notes with hints of what you'll do to be a great mom, and stick them around the house. Affirmations to consider if you **fear your ability to be the best mom** possible include:

- I intend to be a great mother. Even if I make mistakes, I'll still do my best for my baby.
- I'm confident that I'll be a wonderful mom.
- I'll be the mother I've always wanted to be.
- I was specially chosen to parent this baby, and I'll do my best to honor this gift.
- I'll instinctively know my baby's needs, and I'll meet them with love.
- I know how to care for my baby.
- I'll make the best decisions for my baby.

The **fear of an unhealthy baby** can be calmed

with a visualization of your baby developing from an embryo to a full baby. Try these affirmations if you're worried about your baby's health:

- My baby will be healthy and strong.
- My baby is beautiful and full of life.
- My baby is developing perfectly.
- My baby is growing just the way they are supposed to.
- My body can grow a healthy baby.

Worrying about gaining weight or losing it after birth can be conquered if you visualize yourself glowing from pregnancy. Visualize yourself exercising to keep your weight under control. These affirmations can be used if you're worried about weight issues:

- My belly is gorgeous.
- My body nourishes my baby.
- I'm proud of my pregnant body and big bump.
- I embrace the changes to my body as it grows and gives my baby what they need.
- I'm proud and excited to grow my baby inside my body.

Visualizing your baby as a complete being just before birth can help you beat the **fear of miscarriage**. Use these affirmations if you're worried about miscarriage:

- My baby is safe within my womb.
- My body knows how to care for my baby's needs.
- My body was designed to carry my baby.
- My body accepts my baby, and I'm looking forward to meeting him/her.

You can visualize a table filled with all the nutritious foods if you **fear not eating the right stuff**. You can also visualize your baby receiving nutritious food in your belly. These affirmations can help you:

- The food I eat nourishes me and my baby.
- I'll choose nutritious foods to help my baby grow.
- I only want the best nutrition for my baby.

Preterm labor fears can be eased with a visualization of you holding your full-term baby after birth. You can also use these affirmations:

- My baby will be born at the perfect time.
- My baby knows when the time is right, and I can't wait to meet them.
- My baby is developing at the right pace, and they will come when they're ready.

For **general pregnancy anxieties**, you can try some of these affirmations:

- I'm lucky to be growing my baby inside of me.
- Being a mother is a wonderful opportunity for which I'm thankful.
- My baby can feel how much I love them.
- I choose to appreciate every moment of my pregnancy, even when it's hard.
- I'm strong and confident, and I can meet the challenges that come with pregnancy.
- My connection to my baby grows deeper by the day.
- I'm blessed to become a mother.

- I have boundless love for my baby, and they can feel it.

Start taking control of your thought patterns and self-talk. You owe it to yourself and your baby to be excited about this journey, especially if you planned it for a long time. There's nothing more precious than the bond between a mother and child, and pregnancy is merely a stepping stone to get you there. Smile more and realize that worries will only make the journey less enjoyable.

9

STEP 9: ON YOUR MARKS, GET SET, AND RELAX! BE PREPARED OR BE SQUARED

*P*reparing for your baby's arrival can calm the tide of anxiety by removing the uncertainty and unpreparedness factor. Feeling unprepared for something important almost always makes us feel worried and anxious. When you feel prepared, you'll excitedly await your baby, knowing that you are ready. Being prepared for each trimester during pregnancy can also help you bond better with your baby, and it's a great way for dad to get in on the action. You'll both be deeply connected to the baby when you're planning your way forward. Moreover, the fear of not making it on time when the baby comes, eating the wrong foods, and the baby's overall health will be reduced when you're in charge of the little things you can control. Step nine will remind you about what needs to be prepared in each trimester, so you can feel ready and able to welcome your sweet baby.

First Trimester

The first three months of pregnancy is a time of uncertainty, so preparing for what has to be done can certainly remove the fear of the unknown and leave you more relaxed and ready to take charge of your pregnancy. Chances are that something hilarious might even happen in your first 12 weeks. Between morning sickness and cravings, you'll probably have stories to tell. I recall a craving that sent my poor husband all over town for two hours in the middle of the night. Fortunately, it was an edible craving. Sometimes, we get a little pica brain and crave objects that can't be eaten, such as cardboard and dryer fluff. Please do not feed these cravings. Speak to your doctor about them before trying to use Dr. Google to figure out why you're craving oddities. Turning to Google for medical advice is like asking a toddler what stocks you should invest in. Parenting websites are great as long as you can see some credentials or you're taking advice from positive moms, but stay away from the online medical realm because misinformation is abundant.

Anyway, my husband was highly supportive, which was probably due to our struggle to conceive, so we shared a deep appreciation for our unborn baby. We still had fears, and they were probably wilder than most expectant parents, but we were a team. When I said I needed Reese's chocolate ice cream, my husband knew I needed it. We drove from one store to another, and each store only had plain chocolate ice cream to which I would have to add separate Reese's cups. No, I craved the ice cream with the cups already inside, and I was determined I was going to get it. Between pinching my bladder and the random bursts of irritation common with pregnancy hormones, we found the target after two hours.

The night didn't end there, though. Pinching my bladder for so long wasn't a good idea, but my husband had a friend who lived on that side of town. At about midnight, we were knocking some poor guy awake so I could use his bathroom. The friend was thankfully understanding, and by the time we made it home, I was drinking my ice cream from the tub. Pregnancy brain also doesn't always allow for logic, so I didn't think about whether the ice cream could last. However, the night was a great memory that makes us laugh today.

Nonetheless, the first trimester is when you're setting up shop for an improved lifestyle. Ice cream is allowed, but only when the cravings really drive you to it. Pregnant women don't have to avoid treats altogether; you just have to eat them as sparingly as possible.

These are the things you should be preparing in the first 12 weeks:

- Book your first pregnancy confirmation appointment or prenatal visit with your doctor. You should also choose an OB-GYN, midwife, or doula if you haven't yet.
- Design a budget for your baby-related purchases in later pregnancy. Try to save as much money as you can now, so you can purchase all necessary baby items later. The budget should start right away to promote savings, and you can use the zero-based system, which means every dollar and cent must be allocated to a budget entry. This way, you won't be spending excess money if you're planning your

savings, expenses, medical insurance, and daily expenses. It helps to have a monthly budget for entertainment as well. Boredom leads to people spending money that was allocated elsewhere.

- Check your hospital insurance coverage and how many doctors visits it covers. You don't want insurance surprises later in pregnancy. This will only cause unnecessary anxiety, but knowing what your insurance covers can reduce the stress.

- Look for a good prenatal yoga class. Remember to make sure it has discussion times, a qualified instructor, and a positive atmosphere.

- Speak to your doctor about an exercise plan, set it up, and start following it.

- Design weekly meal plans that include all the nutritious foods you enjoy. You can create four different weekly plans and alternate between them to prevent nutritional boredom. Write down recipes you enjoy, and try some new ingredients. You can also change your meal plans as your stomach guides you. Some foods will be okay today and terrible tomorrow. Be flexible with the changes.

- Purchase a pregnancy journal, or use printable templates. Start writing every day.
- Plan a fun way to tell your friends and relatives about the pregnancy. Dads-to-be must also be involved. One idea is to invite your closest friends and relatives over while you stage the house with hints. Hang a onesie in the bathroom, put a bun in the oven, and put some baby wipes on the table instead of hand wipes. Hang a few booties from the flower arrangement, and put some baby-shaped cookies on the table. Put enough hints around the home, and then just wait for someone to say something. Have a camera handy for the reactions when someone finally notices your clues.

Second Trimester

The second trimester will be a busy one, so you need to prepare a few things before diving into the third trimester where everything slows down. I suffered terribly from pregnancy brain in the second trimester, and combining pregnancy brain with the list of to-dos made me think it should be called Jumanji level two. I knew my belly was only going to grow bigger, and I wouldn't have much time or energy to stand cooking for hours in the third level of Jumanji, so I started preparing frozen meals to store safely in airtight glass containers. Let's face it, some days toward the end of your pregnancy, you'll be thankful that you prepared so well. Just be sure to research how long you can freeze certain foods before cooking up a storm. Invite a friend to help out, and make it a fun social event also.

During my flurry of cooking, I ended up with another memorable story. I wanted to bake a fresh loaf of whole-wheat bread because the smell that fills a home is like no other. I wanted to surprise my husband when he returned from work, so I jumped into my recipe book. I found one with cranberries and nuts added, and I was kneading my dough by hand. Finally, I placed it in a baking tray and set the timer. I went off to the living room to kick my feet up while my bread baked. The excitement and mouth-watering started when I heard the timer, and off I went to the kitchen. Upon opening the oven, I was shocked to see my bread was gone! Who came into my home so fast and stole my bread? Suddenly, I realized I couldn't smell my bread, either. Who dared take my bread? My husband would be home any minute!

It was only the next day that I found my bread. Somehow, my pregnancy brain thought it would bake better in the freezer. I couldn't control my laughter when I found the frozen bread pan. My husband was already home, and I think that's the best laugh we've had in years. Anyway, it's time to prepare what needs to be done in the second trimester.

These are the things you should prepare:

- Book your ultrasound. Seeing your baby in detail for the first time will melt your heart.
- Start shopping for maternity clothes, including nursing bras, pajamas, and pads if you're going to breastfeed.
- Sign up for Lamaze or childbirth classes to start familiarizing yourself with realistic expectations and methods to reduce discomfort.
- Start attending prenatal yoga if you haven't already.

- Book your gestational diabetes test at 24 weeks, so you can have peace of mind about the fears related to the condition. Don't panic if you test positive for gestational diabetes. Your doctor will help you keep it under control. Follow their advice, and you'll be doing the best you can. However, if you test negative, just keep eating mostly the right foods, and keep your weight gain steady.

- Start researching the best furniture for your baby, such as a stroller, car seat, and crib (the big purchases). Research the safety features of each as well. It's not about buying the trendiest one. It's about knowing that your baby has the best and safest you can give him/her.

- Sit down with your partner, and create your birth plan. Remember that it may change, and that's okay because it will only change if it's in the baby's best interests. Once you have your plan in hand, you can also discuss it with your doula, midwife, or OB-GYN.

- Tour birth centers if you want to look at various options. Some women opt for water births, and others prefer the traditional hospital birth. It's a good idea to tour all the options you're considering, in case your mind changes before the time.

- Start purchasing your newborn clothes, diapers, toiletries, and blankets. You'll need onesies, booties, newborn hats, non-scratch mitts, rompers, sweaters, and gentle baby laundry detergent. You'll also need diapers, baby wipes, diaper lotion, shampoo, and hooded towels. You can also get baby nail clippers, a thermometer, and a first aid kit. Baby shopping is exciting, apart from the money you have to spend, but that's what the savings were for.

- Plan your route to the birthing center or hospital you chose. It may help to have your partner as the designated driver or someone else close by.

- Start preparing for your departure from work by catching up on your projects and having training information ready for your replacement.

- Start stocking your freezer with prepared meals and meats. Please don't put bread dough in the freezer instead of the oven, but prepped meals will be handy soon.

- Plan your maternity leave. Your doctor will give you a due date, but know that due dates are an estimate. I doubt many babies are born on the predicted day, so try to work at least part-time as long into your pregnancy as is safe. You'll get tired and have to slow down at work, but you'll want to spend more time with your baby once they arrive.

Third Trimester

Reaching the third trimester is both tiring and exciting. Your body has to carry additional weight now, but the excitement comes from knowing your baby will be here soon. Your hormones will likely be all over the place, and that's fine because it's expected. Again, people are more understanding of moms-to-be than you think. It's okay to laugh and cry at the same time, which you'll probably experience at some point. It's okay to feel sad and happy at the same time. Emotional confusion comes with the territory of pregnancy hormones. Never feel bad about the way you feel. You may want to stay away from movies about puppies, babies, and anything cute or romantic if you're afraid of crying. Otherwise, have a box of tissues handy as you let it all out.

A close friend and her husband decided to decorate the nursery during her third trimester. She was in charge of choosing the color for the walls, and her husband would be the painter. Obviously, it's not safe for expectant mothers to paint the nursery. Anyway, you'll be surprised at how many shades of the same color exist. After deep pondering, she chose a shade of pink called lemonade. It looked so pretty on the color chart, and her husband was so happy to show her his hard work when he was done. She walked into the room and was utterly horrified, as she hated the color. On the second try, she chose a shade called blush. Her exhausted husband took her back into the room only to get the same reaction. I'm sure he was impatient at this stage, but he was a supportive man, so she then chose another shade called crepe. Finally, her husband, with his entire week gone to painting the nursery, took her in for another look.

At last, it was finally the right pink. She was blessed with a great husband who put up with her hormonal indecisiveness. His support was only recognized after having their baby when my dear friend realized that the lemonade, blush, and crepe shades of pink all looked exactly the same. Her poor husband sacrificed an entire week while getting pink paint in his hair. Nonetheless, these are the things you want to prepare in the third trimester:

- Decorate your nursery, and move the baby's furniture into place. Make sure you aren't painting because it's not good for the baby, but know that your decisiveness may be affected right now. That's also okay. You can always change something later.

- Start detoxifying your home. Remove the BPA plastics with recycling numbers one, three, six, and seven if you haven't already. Replace these with glass containers. Stop using pesticides and herbicides in your garden because you could bring them into your home. A vacuum cleaner with a high-efficiency particulate air (HEPA) filter is great at removing the dust mites from your home, and start using vinegar to clean surfaces instead of commercial cleaners. A natural cleaner for any surface is one-part white vinegar with one-part water in a spray bottle. Wash your baby's clothing with baby laundry detergent, and use white vinegar to soften it before their arrival. You should also avoid using air fresheners and any cleaning product with glycol ethers. Instead, water down some lavender essential oil in a spray bottle to freshen your home.

- Tour birth centers if you haven't yet.

- Schedule a group B strep test between weeks 35 and 37. This is an inexpensive test that ensures you don't pass the common streptococcus bacteria to your baby during delivery.

- Purchase a book about breastfeeding, or sign up for a breastfeeding class/support group, if you are planning to breastfeed. Many groups don't require advanced enrolment.

- Stock up on nipple pads.

- Finish buying the baby items like onesies, nail clippers, booties, blankets, toiletries, diapers, baby mittens, and the "going home" outfit.

- Choose a pediatrician if that's an option for you. You can get referrals from trusted and positive mom friends, and you're allowed to interview a few until you find the one you like.

- Install your baby's car seat, and have it checked for safety.

- Pack your hospital bag if you haven't done so already. Your pre-packed bag should include your birth plan, soft bathrobe, socks to keep your feet warm during labor, and slippers for comfortable walks around the delivery ward. Indeed, you'll be encouraged to walk around during the early stages of labor, which helps with pain and can speed labor up a bit. You should also pack lip balm as your lips may dry, body lotion for a gentle massage from your co-parent, and a spray bottle of water to use to cool down during labor. You'll need comfortable pillows, an eye mask, earplugs, and some entertainment for those slow times between contractions. You'll also need heavy-duty maternity pads, nightgowns, nursing bras, toiletries, and underwear for after the delivery. Don't forget your phone and charger, reference books, snacks, and drinks. Your hospital bag needs a few essentials for the baby, too. Pack diapers, onesies, wipes, blankets, booties, the going-home outfit, and the basic toiletries you'll need. Please add nail clippers and mitts for your baby, or they'll scratch their faces with those sharp little nails. I know this from first-hand experience. My daughter scratched up her sweet little cheeks her first day on this earth, and she still bears the scars to this day.

- Have your home cleaned toward the end of your third trimester, so you and your baby can have less to worry about, more time to create memories, and restful times to bond.

Being prepared for your trimesters can make this journey as enjoyable as it should be. Don't see the preparation lists as chores, either. Turn them into fun activities, especially shopping for baby supplies. Keep your options open because your hormones will change your mind when you least expect it, and make sure you know what to expect with your insurance and birthing centers. Now, you have control over the things you can control.

CONCLUSION

Pregnancy fears and worries are very common, and some of them won't even seem reasonable once your baby arrives. A plate that should be full of happy memories, kicks that remind you to smile, and ultrasound photo collages that make your heart skip a beat is instead filled with all the wrong things for many newly pregnant and first-time moms-to-be. From worrying about your feet getting wider to wondering if you'll be able to breastfeed your baby, pregnancy sure throws new moms-to-be a curveball if they allow it to. We can't worry about everything on this journey because fear is not the right motivator to sustain the best pregnancy we can. Pride, joy, and excitement are the better motivators.

The fear of being a bad mother, eating the wrong foods, and morning sickness will only take the happiness out of your journey and leave you with a pile of anxiety and stress, both of which aren't good for your baby. It's not good for the baby when you worry about what you should expect during labor, especially not if you're listening to a bunch of ladies who see the negative side of everything. Fear isn't healthy if you keep worrying about birth defects, instead of leading a better pregnancy journey that crushes the risks. Fear leads to doubts, and soon enough, you're struggling with your pregnancy.

The only truth about fear is that it can create phantom symptoms, which may increase the risks of unwanted outcomes. Stop fearing preterm labor and c-sections unless a doctor is about to rush you into surgery. Think about it this way. Imagine fearing a tree falling onto your house, and because of that fear, you eventually decide to cut it down. Now, your house is baking in the sun every day, but the tree, that was deeply rooted in the ground, is now gone. Sometimes, we fear what may never manifest, and pregnancy concerns are in that category. The risk of complications is so low that you're cutting a tree down before it falls, which it may never do. Without shade, your home doesn't seem so wonderful anymore.

Without taking control of what you can control in pregnancy, your journey might be filled with worry and stress in the place of comforting shade, if the shade represents a deeper connection to your baby and happy memories. Not knowing what to do is one thing, but choosing to be anxious instead of learning what can be controlled is another thing altogether. This is your journey. It's about your baby growing inside of you. Don't let anxiety steal your experience. You know the facts about complications now, so you can stop asking negative Nancy to share her stories.

You know what to expect during labor, so don't allow fictional movies to horrify you when real-life might be so different. And who knows? You might just be like my friend Jess who was fortunate enough to sleep through labor. Listen to stories from women who laughed so hard during labor that they pushed their babies out. Listen to the moms who share the emotional epiphany when their babies are born. Start educating yourself more about the expectations you should have, and stop reading stories about Amber whose water broke in the dairy section of the supermarket. Stop feeling ashamed of your body when it's the most beautiful figure you can ever wear.

Start exercising, attending prenatal yoga, and eating foods that keep you and your baby in pristine health. Start sleeping the way a pregnant woman deserves, and don't let yourself ignore your needs. You're pregnant. You're allowed to feel happy, sad, tired, angry, hungry, and confused at the same time. Anyone who comments on your hormonal changes is obviously not a mother. And sure, have your tub of ice cream from two towns over when you feel like it. Mix foods that make no sense, and stop caring about other people's opinions. Just stick to your nutritious foods most of the time. Go swimming every day if you want. As much as you imagine your big belly pulling you down, it won't.

Meet people who encourage you to be happy during this time, and allow them to show you how wildly inaccurate movies have made your expectations of birth. Go and learn the breathing techniques and position changes that may make the birth easier. Take charge of how you bond with your baby, and encourage your partner to do the same. The memories you can create during your bonding exercises with your unborn baby can last a lifetime. Imagine seeing your child's face one day as you hand them the letter you wrote while pregnant. Give it to them as a special gift when they're expecting one day in the distant future.

Take back control of your mindset so your thoughts and emotions can mostly belong to your reasoning self again. Indeed, pregnancy brain will interfere from time to time. You may find underwear in the microwave and chicken in the washing machine, but that's okay. It happens, and it makes for great memories. Planning and preparing for each trimester can help you with pregnancy brain. It can also help you soothe the anxieties about being pregnant and what you're supposed to do. There are many aspects of pregnancy you can control, and you know what they are now. There's nothing left to fear. That's it. As long as you lead a lifestyle conducive to your baby's development, that's all you can control.

I feel a weight lifted when I help another mom-to-be. I know where you are, and I know what it feels like. I'd also love to know how this advice is working for you. I welcome you to leave a comment or review to let me know how your journey changed. It may also help other new moms-to-be find positive information that could actually help them. Every mom-to-be whole-heartedly deserves to travel this journey without anxiety and stress. Every mom-to-be deserves a connected and unexplainably joyful pregnancy. My last piece of advice to you is this: Go into the world, and show them how pregnant women should thrive in their journeys. Be the example that sets a trend for everyone else.

10

REFERENCES

*A*pta Club. (2019, June 11). *Reasons to talk to your baby before birth.* Aptamil™. https://www.aptaclub.co.uk/pregnancy/bonding-and-development/reasons-to-talk-to-your-baby-before-birth.html

Baby Centre. (2021, March). *10 ways to bond with your baby bump.* Baby Centre UK. https://www.babycentre.co.uk/a1049630/10-ways-to-bond-with-your-baby-bump

Bacaro, V., Benz, F., Pappaccogli, A., De Bartolo, P., Johann, A. F., Palagini, L., Lombardo, C., Feige, B., Riemann, D., & Baglioni, C. (2020). Interventions for sleep problems during pregnancy: A systematic review. *Sleep Medicine Reviews, 50,* 101234. https://doi.org/10.1016/j.smrv.2019.101234

Ben-Joseph, E. P. (2017). *Eating during pregnancy (for parents).* Kidshealth.org. https://kidshealth.org/en/parents/eating-pregnancy.html

Bhoopalam, P. S., & Watkinson, M. (1991). Babies born before arrival at hospital. *BJOG: An International Journal of Obstetrics and Gynaecology, 98*(1), 57–64. https://doi.org/10.1111/j.1471-0528.1991.tb10312.x

Brainy Quote. (n.d.). *Rodney Dangerfield quotes.* Brainy Quote. https://www.brainyquote.com/quotes/rodney_dangerfield_100124

Campbell, V. R., & Nolan, M. (2016). A qualitative study exploring how the aims, language and actions of yoga for pregnancy teachers may impact upon women's self-efficacy for labour and birth. *Women and Birth, 29*(1), 3–11. https://doi.org/10.1016/j.wombi.2015.04.007

Campbell, V., & Nolan, M. (2019). "It definitely made a difference": A grounded theory study of yoga for pregnancy and women's self-efficacy for labour.

Midwifery, 68, 74–83. https://doi.org/10.1016/j.midw.2018.10.005

Cascio, C. N., O'Donnell, M. B., Tinney, F. J., Lieberman, M. D., Taylor, S. E., Strecher, V. J., & Falk, E. B. (2015). Self-affirmation activates brain systems associated with self-related processing and reward and is reinforced by future orientation. *Social Cognitive and Affective Neuroscience*, 11(4), 621–629. https://doi.org/10.1093/scan/nsv136

CDC. (2020, November 16). *What is stillbirth?* Centers for Disease Control and Prevention. https://www.cdc.gov/ncbddd/stillbirth/facts.html#:~:text=Stillbirth%20affects%20about%201%20in

Cedars Sinai. (2021). *What to expect during your first childbirth*. Cedars-Sinai. https://www.cedars-sinai.org/programs/obstetrics-maternity/delivery/first-time.html

Condie, N. (2020, September 8). *Easing miscarriage worries during the first 12 weeks of pregnancy*. Cache Valley Women's Center. https://www.cvwomenscenter.com/blog/easing-miscarriage-worries/

De Bellefonds, C. (2019, April 26). *8 common pregnancy sleep problems*. What to Expect. https://www. whattoexpect.com/pregnancy/sleep-solutions/ pregnancy-sleep-problems-solutions/

De Bellefonds, C., & Rebarber, A. (2021, March 16). *What's the best sleeping position during pregnancy?* What to Expect. https://www.whattoexpect.com/ pregnancy/sleep-solutions/pregnancy-sleep-positions/

De Campos, E. A., Narchi, N. Z., & Moreno, G. (2020). Meanings and perceptions of women regarding the practice of yoga in pregnancy: A qualitative study. *Complementary Therapies in Clinical Practice*, 39, 101099. https://doi.org/10.1016/j. ctcp.2020.101099

Doi, S. A. R., Furuya-Kanamori, L., Toft, E., Musa, O. A. H., Mohamed, A. M., Clark, J., & Thalib, L. (2020). Physical activity in pregnancy prevents gestational diabetes: A meta-analysis. *Diabetes Research and Clinical Practice*, 168(), 108371. https://doi.org/10.1016/j.diabres.2020.108371

Dreisbach, S. (2015, July 14). *Top 14 pregnancy fears (and why you shouldn't worry)*. Parents; https://

www.parents.com/pregnancy/complications/health-and-safety-issues/top-pregnancy-fears/

Felder, J. N., Epel, E. S., Neuhaus, J., Krystal, A. D., & Prather, A. A. (2020). Efficacy of digital cognitive behavioral therapy for the treatment of insomnia symptoms among pregnant women. *JAMA Psychiatry.* https://doi.org/10.1001/jamapsychiatry.2019.4491

Fernandez, E. (2019, July 8). How to write your own positive pregnancy affirmations. Elayna Fernandez: The Positive Mom. https://www.thepositivemom.com/write-positive-pregnancy-affirmations

Goddijn, M., & Leschot, N. J. (2000). Genetic aspects of miscarriage. *Best Practice & Research Clinical Obstetrics & Gynaecology,* 14(5), 855–865. https://doi.org/10.1053/beog.2000.0124

Goldner, D. (2015, June 11). *Bonding with baby-to-be.* Parents. https://www.parents.com/pregnancy/my-life/preparing-for-baby/bonding-with-baby-to-be/

Haring, M., Smith, J. E., Bodnar, D., Misri, S., Little, R. M., & Ryan, D. (2013, February). *Coping with anxiety during pregnancy and following the birth.* BC Mental Health and Addiction Services. http://www.bcmhsus.ca/Documents/coping-with-anxiety-during-pregnancy-an   d-following-the-birth.pdf

Haupt, A. (2021). *How to have a happier, healthier, smarter baby.* US News & World Report; https:// health.usnews.com/health-news/family-health/ childrens-health/articles/2010/10/19/how-to-have-a-happier-healthier-smarter-baby

Health Link BC. (2016, June 14). *Healthy eating guidelines for food safety during pregnancy.* Health Link BC. https://www.healthlinkbc.ca/healthy-eating/pregnancy-food-safety

Hecht, A. (2006, December). *Exercise during pregnancy.* WebMD; https://www.webmd.com/baby/guide/exercise-during-pregnancy#1

Korneva, J. (2018, August 8). *Bonding with that bump: 20 ways moms can bond with their baby during pregnancy.* Moms. https://www.moms.com/bonding-with-that-bump-20-ways-moms-can-bond-with-their-baby-during-pregnancy/

Kubala, J., & Bjarnadottir, A. (2018, July 18). *11 foods and beverages to avoid during pregnancy.* Healthline; https://www.healthline.com/nutrition/ 11-foods-to-avoid-during-pregnancy

Lerner, H., & Snyder, C. (2020, August 30). *How to gain control of your life from pregnancy stress.* Verywell Family. https://www.verywellfamily.com/tips-coping-with-stress-during-pregnancy-3520997

Liles, M. (2019, December 23). *100 pregnancy quotes for moms-to-be that describe what being pregnant is all about.* Parade: Entertainment, Recipes, Health, Life, Holidays. https://parade.com/971665/ marynliles/pregnancy-quotes/

Marcin, A., & Dishman, K. (2016, May 23). *7 tips to ease anxiety during pregnancy.* Healthline. https:// www.healthline.com/health/pregnancy/anxiety-coping-tips#symptoms

Marcin, A., & Nwadike, V. R. (2020, May 20). *After your water breaks, how long can baby survive?* Healthline. https://www.healthline.com/health/ pregnancy/after-water-breaks-how-long-baby-can-survive#:~:text=When%20this%20sac% 20breaks%2C%20it

Miles, K., & Mindell, J. (2020, November 10). *The basics of good sleep during pregnancy.* Baby Center. https://www.babycenter.com/pregnancy/your-body/the-basics-of-good-sleep-during-pregnancy_7820

Mooventhan, A. (2019). A comprehensive review on scientific evidence-based effects (including adverse effects) of yoga for normal and high-risk pregnancy-related health problems. *Journal of Bodywork and Movement Therapies, 23,* 721–727. https://doi.org/10.1016/j.jbmt.2019.03.005

Newman, T., & Butler, N. (2017, May 24). *Pregnancy diet: What to eat and what to avoid.* Medical News Today. https://www.medicalnewstoday.com/articles/246404#rules

Nierenberg, C. (2018, January 10). *Pregnancy diet & nutrition: What to eat, what not to eat.* Live Science; https://www.livescience.com/45090-pregnancy-diet.html

Orlans, M. (2015, April 25). *Are unborn babies aware?* LinkedIn. https://www.linkedin.com/pulse/unborn-babies-aware-michael-orlans/

Pregnancy: Birth and Baby. (2019). *Bonding with your baby during pregnancy*. Pregnancy: Birth and Baby; https://www.pregnancybirthbaby.org.au/bonding-with-your-baby-during-pregnancy

Public Health Scotland. (2020, September 22). *Attachment and bonding during pregnancy*. NHS Inform Scotland. https://www.nhsinform.scot/ready-steady-baby/pregnancy/relationships-and-wellbeing-in-pregnancy/attachment-and-bonding-during-pregnancy

Rai, R., & Regan, L. (2006). Recurrent miscarriage. *The Lancet*, 368(9535), 601–611. https://doi.org/10.1016/s0140-6736(06)69204-0

Regan, L., & Rai, R. (2000). Epidemiology and the medical causes of miscarriage. *Best Practice & Research Clinical Obstetrics & Gynaecology*, 14(5), 839–854. https://doi.org/10.1053/beog.2000.0123

Ross-White, A. (2017, October 17). *Two simple ways to lower odds of stillbirth*. CNN. https://edition.cnn.com/2017/10/16/health/prevent-stillbirth-kicks-back-sleep-partner

Schnabolk, L. C. (2020, December). *Top pregnancy fears: When to worry and when to let go.* The Bump. https://www.thebump.com/a/top-pregnancy-fears

Sorgen, C. (n.d.). *Bonding with baby before birth.* WebMD. https://www.webmd.com/baby/features/bonding-with-baby-before-birth#1

Tarkan, L. (2018, November 19). *Top pregnancy fears you can feel better about.* Parents. https://www.parents.com/pregnancy/my-life/top-pregnancy-fears-you-can-feel-better-about/

Taylor, M., & Wu, J. (2020, May 20). *8 best foods for pregnant women.* What to Expect. https://www.whattoexpect.com/pregnancy/eating-well/week-11/big-nutrition-small-packages.aspx

Traylor, C. S., Johnson, J. D., Kimmel, M. C., & Manuck, T. A. (2020). Effects of psychological stress on adverse pregnancy outcomes and nonpharmacologic approaches for reduction: An expert review. *American Journal of Obstetrics & Gynecology MFM,* 2(4), 100229. https://doi.org/10.1016/j.ajogmf.2020.100229

University of Cambridge. (2018, June 12). *Mother's attitude to baby during pregnancy may have implica-*

tions for child's development. Science Daily. https://www.sciencedaily.com/releases/2018/06/180612105757.htm

Victoria State Government. (2012). *Pregnancy and diet.* Victoria State Government. https://www.betterhealth.vic.gov.au/health/healthyliving/pregnancy-and-diet

Vismara, L., Rollè, L., Agostini, F., Sechi, C., Fenaroli, V., Molgora, S., Neri, E., Prino, L. E., Odorisio, F., Trovato, A., Polizzi, C., Brustia, P., Lucarelli, L., Monti, F., Saita, E., & Tambelli, R. (2016). Perinatal parenting stress, anxiety, and depression outcomes in first-time mothers and fathers: A 3- to 6- months postpartum follow-up study. *Frontiers in Psychology, 7.* https://doi.org/10.3389/fpsyg.2016.00938

WebMD. (n.d.). *Pregnancy fitness, your best moves before baby arrives.* WebMD. https://www.webmd.com/baby/ss/slideshow-pregnancy-fitness-moves

WebMD. (2002a, May 27). *Eating right when pregnant.* WebMD; https://www.webmd.com/baby/guide/eating-right-when-pregnant#1

WebMD. (2002b, May 27). *Gain weight safely during your pregnancy*. WebMD; https://www.webmd.com/baby/guide/healthy-weight-gain#1

Wheatley, S. (2018, November 15). *Why bonding during pregnancy matters*. Psychreg. https://www.psychreg.org/bonding-pregnancy/

Made in the USA
Monee, IL
08 March 2023